"*The Truth About Herpes* is more than a resource for patients with herpes. It is a necessity. It has been written with all the information a doctor should know about this important disease but it has also been written with compassion and in a language every patient will understand."

> *Dr. Michael V. Reitano*
> *Editor-in-Chief of Sexual Health Magazine*
> *Director of the Herpes Advice Center*
> *Attending physician New York University*

"The new edition of *The Truth About Herpes* is an excellent addition to the literature and provides a comprehensive account of the clinical features, new diagnostic methods, advances in treatment, and psychological implications of genital herpes. All patients with genital herpes should read this book."

> *Dr. Adrian Mindel*
> *Academic Unit of Sexual Health Medicine*
> *The University of Sydney*
> *The University of New South Wales*

"This new edition of Dr. Sacks's book continues its tradition of service to patients by providing cutting-edge information in a reader-friendly style."

> *Dr. S.L. Spruance*
> *Professor of Medicine*
> *School of Medicine*
> *University of Utah*

"I wanted to write a note of thanks and appreciation. The past eight weeks have changed my life considerably and because of you, I am learning to cope. It's hard to imagine that the course of one evening can change so much in one's life. I've done the "guilt and feeling sorry for myself" numbers and now through you and your book—it's time to accept, learn and live. I related to so much in your book (as I'm sure everyone in similar predicaments does) that I almost felt it was written for me. You put things in simple terms and with humour in appropriate places...The time and effort you put into your work reflects the kind of man you are. We, as patients, have a lot to thank you for, both as a professional doctor and as a very understanding man. Again—thank you so much for everything."

> *L.W.*
> *Vancouver*

The Truth
About Herpes

4th edition

Stephen L. Sacks, MD, FRCPC

Professor
Department of Pharmacology and Therapeutics, Faculty of Medicine
University of British Columbia

Founder and Medical Director
Viridae Clinical Sciences, Inc.

Gordon Soules Book Publishers Ltd.
West Vancouver, Canada
Seattle, U.S.

Canadian Cataloguing in Publication Data

> Sacks, Stephen L., 1948–
> The truth about herpes
>
> Includes bibliographical references and index.
> ISBN 0-919574-66-1
>
> 1. Herpes simplex.   I. Title.
> RC147.H6S22 1997   616.95'18   C97-910056-9

Published in Canada by
Gordon Soules Book Publishers Ltd.
1354-B Marine Drive
West Vancouver, BC V7T 1B5
(604) 922-6588 or (604) 688-5466
Fax: (604) 688-5442
E-mail: books@gordonsoules.com
Web site: http://www.gordonsoules.com

Published in the United States by
Gordon Soules Book Publishers Ltd.
620—1916 Pike Place
Seattle, WA 98101
(604) 922-6588 or (604) 688-5466
Fax: (604) 688-5442
E-mail: books@gordonsoules.com
Web site: http://www.gordonsoules.com

We would like to acknowledge the contribution of Verdant Press in the publishing of this and previous editions of this book.

Design by Harry Bardal Design
Printed and bound in Canada by Best Book Manufacturers

To Anne,
Marika,
Adrian and Rebecca,
Krystyna, Richard,
and the memory of my
father, Leon

Contents

Acknowledgments

I would like to express thanks to my coworkers, past and present, at the Herpes Clinic and the Infectious Diseases Laboratory at the University of British Columbia, who have made this book possible. Recently, we moved our clinical research projects to Viridae Clinical Sciences, Inc. in Vancouver. These individuals have provided counseling, administered research, worked with cell cultures and new drugs, and coped with personal crises and funding fluctuations. Without them, there would be no experience to share with you. They are Mike Ashe, Maureen Barfoot, Marion Barker, Gwen Bebault, Danielle Blackburn, Pam Brewis, Leigh Brooker, P. Lynn Buhler, Lynda Clelland, Susan Crooks, Paul Crosson, Shaun Culham, Kim Davies, Joyce Diggins, Sandra Doll, Dr. Pat Doyle, Natalie Dzenkiw, Morrie Eaman, Rebecca Fox, Denise Galipeau, Paula Galloway, Dr. Suzanne Garland, Dr. Greg Grant, Kelly Grant, Terri Grant, Gabriella Guerrato, Patti Hansinger, April Hughes, Charlene Hutchinson, Lisa Jenkinson, Michael Jensen, Rita Jervis, Barbara Johnson, Susan Kingsley, Roger Kong, Philip Lai, Michael Lau, Thinh Le, Laurel Lemchuk-Favel, Andrew Lesperance, Paul Levendusky, Rob McAllister, Carys McDougall, Maggie Macintosh, Maureen Maher, Dr. Wafeeq Mahmoud, Lianne Martin, Ken Morrison, Herma Neyndorff, Megan O'Conner, Joanne Powell, Susan Rayner, Bruce Rennie, Nancy Ruedy, Marika Sacks, Dr. Joseph Sasadeusz, Jean Schwartz, Rashieda Slamang, Leo Smyrnis, Danielle Soulodre, Dale Stromberg, Darlene Taylor, Lori Teather, Marybelle Tingley, Stephanie Tofield, Diljit Uppal, Geraldine Walsh, Jim Wanklin, Elda Wilson, and Chong Ze-Teh. Harry Bardal, Marguerite Drummond, and Bruce Stewart did the illustrations.

Neonatal infection photographs were kindly supplied by Dr. Suzanne Garland. Astra Pharmaceuticals and the Canadian Public Health Association helped to get the first edition off the ground. Burroughs Wellcome Inc. assisted with the distribution of the third edition of this book to thousands of practicing health care professionals. John Vavricka of SmithKline Beecham Pharmaceuticals kindly offered several of the color graphics and electron micrographs for this edition which were created by several talented scientists and graphic artists at that company. Both SmithKline Beecham Pharmaceuticals and Glaxo Wellcome, Inc. have been very helpful in making the availability of this book known to people with herpes. Bruce Wilson worked for me as editor and consultant. Without him, the manuscript simply would never have been completed. Harry Bardal designed and guided the production of the book's new cover. Marika Sacks served as editor, added the chapter quotations, advised on content, and translated many of my thoughts into coherent English. I thank you all.

Most of all, I thank my patients, who have given their blood, their pictures, and their cultures for my teaching and research. They have given me the reasons to teach about herpes and to seek new methods for treatment. They have shared with me their secrets, their pains, their joys, and their thanks.

Preface

Before you begin this book, I'd like you to know a bit about me so you can decide how to interpret what I am calling here the truth about herpes. I am a physician and clinical scientist trained in the area of viral diseases. Since coming to the University of British Columbia as an Assistant Professor in 1980, I have devoted much of my professional life to the study of genital herpes and the care of patients with genital herpes. That same year, I founded the Herpes Clinic for the care of patients and research into the causes, prevention, and treatment of genital herpes. I became a full Professor of Medicine in 1990 and, in 1996, moved to the Department of Pharmacology and Therapeutics in order to focus more on treatment. In 1993 I started a company—Viridae Clinical Sciences, Inc.—for the study and care of people with chronic viral diseases. The Herpes Clinic now operates from Viridae.

Over the past decade or so, I have worked extensively with the pharmaceutical industry. I have been involved in the study of virtually all of the candidate or current treatments for genital herpes. As a result, my staff, my laboratory, my university, my company, and/or I myself have, from time to time, provided paid services to U.S. and Canadian government granting agencies and to just about every pharmaceutical company in the herpes treatment business. In the course of my work, I have given lectures on treatments to doctors and frequently provided consultation to companies developing new treatments. Although my collaboration with the pharmaceutical industry keeps me exposed to the latest information on herpes and the many treatments being studied, it also places me in a potential conflict of interest. Throughout the writing of this book, I have taken every step I know of to remain impartial and to provide balance in presenting the results of clinical treatment trials. The needs of the person with herpes is always my first priority. No pharmaceutical company or representative of any company saw or commented on this book or manuscript prior to its publication. I am personally responsible for the book's content.

I have attempted to provide all the latest information available about drug treatments and diagnostic tests, regardless of whether or not a drug or indication has been approved by the FDA. Some of the treatments discussed here are not yet approved for clinical application in the way they have been used in research or reported in this book, and some may never be. The rapid progress of science in this area will render at least some of the information in this book obsolete before you read it. You should never undertake treatment based entirely on this or any other book. Any decision to take prescription medication should be made only after proper advice from your doctor. He or she will be aware of what medication is currently available and what doses are appropriate. Only your doctor can judge whether a particular treatment would be appropriate, safe, and effective for you. This book is intended to be informative and thought-provoking; it is not intended to be used to replace your own physician's care.

Stephen L. Sacks, M.D.
Vancouver, British Columbia.

Introduction to the
Fourth Edition

There is no new cure. There is no permanent solution yet at hand. So why write yet another edition of this book? The chief objectives have not changed. There is a lot to know about having herpes, and the chapters to follow tell all. Since the last edition, there has been an explosion of discovery and new information around the subject. Much of the new information is reassuring and some a bit unsettling. A new technology called polymerase chain reaction (PCR) allows scientists to detect minute quantities of viral DNA from skin swabs. PCR studies of patients with recurrent genital herpes have shown that herpes probably reactivates far more frequently than anyone realized previously. On the other hand, the vast majority of these reactivations are promptly dealt with by the body's own immune system without ever allowing the viral shedding or clinical symptoms to take hold. Clinical studies have also now shown that safe, long-term recurrence reduction is possible. Proper use of medication can drastically reduce both symptomatic and asymptomatic viral shedding. Reducing asymptomatic shedding might also diminish the chances of asymptomatic transmission of herpes simplex virus, although this remains to be proven. Early results suggest that cesarean section might be avoidable in many cases by using acyclovir suppression during the last few weeks of pregnancy (see discussion chapter 6). Antiviral chemotherapy has reached its second generation and studies are under way to determine how much improvement we can identify. Dosing of treatments has become easier, and effectiveness has also improved. Vaccine trials for both prevention and treatment are ongoing although early results with one of the current vaccine candidates have been discouraging. The key issues for most people, though, remain the simple, personal ones. How do I tell my partner I have herpes? How do I avoid transmitting the infection? How do I break this burden of self-imposed secrecy and keep my self-esteem intact? How do I avoid feeling like a victim? How do I get on with my life?

Herpes has also changed over the past decade because of the AIDS epidemic. Research into HIV infection has brought with it new understanding of and new treatments for other viral diseases like herpes. The immune surveillance system that controls herpes in the normal host is diminished in AIDS, so herpes is one of the common problems affecting people with AIDS. But the AIDS epidemic has also meant that safer sex is becoming commonplace. If you are having sexual contact, you should be using safer sex practices. The sad truth, though, is that too many people are still not discussing safer sex or routinely practicing it. Safer sex practices should be considered the normal and usual thing to do until you and your partner have both determined your risks for all STDs including AIDS and until you have both decided to be completely monogamous. New data on genital herpes are also showing that safer sex in conjunction with avoiding intercourse altogether during active phases of infections is the best way to go for herpes prevention.

The past five years have provided lots of new information about the prevention of sexually transmitted herpes and also lots of new information about the prevention of herpes in newborn babies. Acyclovir has now been in general use for nearly fifteen years, and its safety has been remarkable, to date. Under certain circumstances, some physicians have even begun to prescribe acyclovir for chronic suppression in children and pregnant women (see discussion chapter 6). Two new drugs for herpes have been approved by the FDA. New drugs have a major role to play in the treatment of genital herpes. In some cases, though, drug treatment is not very helpful. The right drug used the wrong way can make coping with genital herpes more difficult. This book will help you and your physician through the maze of therapeutic decision-making.

The next generation of drugs for herpes may hold even more promise, and clinical trials are not far off. Scientists have identified some of the gene products of herpes that somehow allow the virus to maintain its latent state. Certain genes allow herpes to become latent, stay latent and not reactivate at all. It is possible, therefore, that specific targets for new chemotherapy will be identified to attempt to prevent reactivation. Today, such products remain on the preclinical drawing boards. Ten years ago, however, there were no such discussions. Ten years from now, new treatments and vaccines will likely be preventing new infection in partners and reducing the problem of herpes recurrences even further. Reversing genetic characteristics of latent herpes to prevent further disease could well be the next step.

Hopes for cures remain alive. In the meantime, new discoveries and old discoveries make treatments much more safe and effective. Use them wisely. You don't need to become celibate or promiscuous in an effort to cope with herpes. Instead, you can stress honesty and be selective in choosing partners on the basis of mutual respect. You can use safer sex practices to avoid the transmission of AIDS, Chlamydia, papillomavirus, gonorrhea, and herpes. You can talk about your herpes assertively and apologize to no one for being clear about what is going on in your own body and for knowing what to do about it. Especially, you don't need to apologize to yourself. You can find out what you need to find out, discuss what you need to discuss, and treat what you need to treat. This book should help you to do all three.

Introduction to the First Edition

If I have herpes, does that make me a sexual leper? Is herpes a sign of the Apocalypse? Is it the wrath of God? A modern day plague? Will I be able to have children if I get it? Will it give me cancer? Is it incurable? Should I become celibate? Should I see a divorce lawyer? Will I go blind? Is this the incurable social disease which deforms babies and causes cancer? These concerns, and many more, are very real ones for the thousands of people whose lives are touched by herpes. The questions are numerous, and they keep coming. Answers are essential.

At the University of British Columbia Herpes Clinic, one of only a handful of its kind in North America, we have seen hundreds of genital herpes sufferers. We have listened carefully to thousands of questions, and done our best to answer them with facts. A glance at the table of contents will give you an idea of what people are asking. The answers are based on current medical knowledge and day-by-day clinical experience.

There is no question that herpes is a growing problem. The number of people affected is increasing at an alarming rate. Unfortunately, misinformation has increased with the growth rate. We do not know just how many people are affected with herpes, but guesses of 500,000 to 1,000,000 new cases in North America per year have been made. These figures are generally based on the number of herpes sufferers who go to clinics which treat sexually transmitted diseases. However, all people with herpes do not necessarily go to such clinics. Family doctors, as well as specialists in dermatology, urology, gynecology, or infectious diseases, are diagnosing and treating herpes. Furthermore, because herpes is not always diagnosed with a standard lab test and because it is not, for physicians, a "notifiable" disease like syphilis or tuberculosis, there are no dependable statistics. During the last decade the number of people seeking medical attention for this problem has increased nearly tenfold. Along with the rise in incidence of genital herpes, there has been a parallel upswing in media attention. Some have suggested that the problem has grown more in print than in victims. While there is an element of truth in this, herpes remains all too real to the person who has it. It is a serious concern to anyone who is or who plans to be sexually active in their life, whether those plans include one lifetime partner or a hundred. Coping with and living a normal life around herpes is a challenge which can be met. To meet the challenge, however, you have to arm yourself with the truth. Unfortunately, the dissemination of useful information has not always been the goal in the current media obsession with the disease. For television and the newspapers, herpes has become a major "news" event—from public affairs shows to the eleven o'clock news, from glossy magazines to hardcore newsmagazines. Such unrelenting public exposure to the problem has actually changed the disease itself. Herpes is no longer just a sexually transmitted infection which requires understanding—it has become a stigma which requires destigmatizing. We are subjected to flashy headlines and frightening stories; home remedies and personal tragedies. Herpes has good selling power but all too often, unfortunately, fear is transmitted in lieu of information.

Television, magazines, and even books wholly devoted to herpes have only rarely dealt with the subject with care. Whether it is the personal anecdotes told at cocktail parties or summarized in seventy printed words next to an ad for perfume, the issues surrounding this common infection have all too often been dealt with in a haphazard fashion. Even the medical profession has had a tough job of it. The time required to inform the patient fully about the problem, explain the details, and answer the questions is not always available in the doctor's office.

Several good organizations have been formed to help provide reliable information about herpes, but unless you're aware that they exist, they can't be of any help. Most of what's in print about herpes avoids the difficult questions, talking about the subject in a superficial way. This book is different. It will take you step by step through the plain facts. Your fears surrounding herpes will be honestly met—nothing, pleasant or unpleasant, is glossed over. Yet the truth has a way of placing fears into perspective. If you are reading this book to learn whether you have herpes—read on. It is important that you do find out, and this book will tell you how to do just that. If you are reading it to find a method for prevention—read on. You may not find a simple answer to the question, but you will know enough to approach prevention intelligently. If you are a physician, you will find the book useful as a tool to help your patients cope with their herpes. It will show you what each person with herpes needs to know in order to live with it.

It is my hope that each person reading this book will realize that herpes is everyone's problem and everyone's concern. Whether you think you have herpes or think that you don't, you should be armed with the truth when you joke about herpes at a party or when you begin your next intimate relationship. You should know the facts before deciding you have never had or never will have this problem. You should know more than you do now before you agree or disagree that herpes may be "the wrath of God." You must learn more before you decide "it will never happen to me."

This book will give you new insight into a growing problem. It is my hope that the misconceptions which result from ignorance will cease to be the single, most important problem about herpes.

1

The Most Important
Questions First

And you want to travel with her,
you want to travel blind
and you know that she can trust you
because you've touched her perfect body
with your mind

—LEONARD COHEN
"Suzanne Takes You Down",
Selected Poems, 1956–1968

Am I contagious between recurrences? Do I have to give up sex?

Medical explanations of herpes are given in the forthcoming chapters. For now, it is most important to know that the virus called *herpes simplex* can exist in two very different states: active, in which the virus is growing on the skin, often forming lesions, and latent, in which the virus is dormant within the nervous system, causing no harm. The latent period is a quiet period that persists for life. From the latent state, the herpes virus may seed a recurrence of an active skin infection.

When your herpes is in the latent state, there is no virus on your skin and you cannot infect your sexual partner. Herpes is only transmitted when active virus on the skin comes into direct contact with the skin of another person who is susceptible. But it is not always possible to know when the virus has reactivated—some infections can go entirely unnoticed. Therefore people with herpes should avoid sore-to-skin contact when obvious skin lesions are present and safer sex should be practiced between episodes—just in case the virus has reactivated without being recognized.

People with herpes must get to know their own recurrence pattern and learn the skills necessary to identify the active periods when the virus is on the skin (see chapter 3). They can then adjust their sexual activity around these times, avoiding sore-to-skin contact during the active phases. Active phases are not made safe by covering a sore with a latex condom.

Often, active herpes infections are mild and not especially bothersome. Every so often, most people with herpes have outbreaks so mild that nothing at all is detected. This no symptoms/no signs recurrence on the skin is called *asymptomatic shedding*—a period of virus reactivation so mild that sores are not detected. A swab taken from the affected area at that time and sent to the laboratory, though, would show that herpes is actively growing on the skin. Thus, it is possible to transmit herpes even though you cannot see a lesion. New data show that suppressive use of antiviral medication—taken continuously twice a day—may reduce the risk of asymptomatic shedding by about 80 percent. Even though asymptomatic shedding occurs less than 5 percent of the time, a person with herpes who is partnered with someone who does not have herpes can take one additional and very effective step toward reducing the risk of transmission: safer sexual practices. The consistent use of latex condoms to prevent direct skin contact during the latent state markedly reduces the chance that an unrecognized recurrence might lead to transmission. In addition, people with herpes should get to know the facts about herpes, so that they can inform their partners assertively and comfortably and be able to explain the risks. Limiting contact to others who have the same infection would accomplish nothing. Furthermore, celibacy would do the world no favor. Indeed, in the long run these extreme measures would do a great deal of harm, both to individuals with herpes and to society at large.

My spouse is my only sexual partner. We've been together for months and I just got herpes. Is my spouse to blame? Has my spouse been unfaithful?

Genital herpes is a sexually transmitted disease. In theory, there is a small possibility of obtaining the infection from another source— for instance, from a warm, moist towel that someone else has just used. In practice, however, for the virus to affect the genitals it must be put *onto* the genitals, and the best way of doing that is via sex. Herpes infections flare up and then heal in a very short cycle, so the virus becomes active, then latent, and then active again. Also, *most* people with genital herpes do not know they have it and never have any symptoms that they identify. Your partner could have been infected in the past and may have had sex with you at the exact moment that he or she had an active infection. There is also the possibility that you have had genital herpes for several years and only just now noticed symptoms. Only very sophisticated laboratory tests can tell the difference between primary and recurrent herpes.

If you have oral sex while either you or your partner are actively shedding virus from the lips or mouth, genital herpes may result. For example, if your partner's mouth came into contact with your genitals, you may have been infected with genital herpes. This can happen if your partner had an active cold sore, a fever blister, or a mouth sore caused by the herpes virus—or even if he or she had no recognized symptoms at all. In fact, 50 to 80 percent of people harbor the virus in a latent state and shed the virus in the mouth during recurrences of active infection.

Herpes simplex causes both mouth and genital herpes. The mouth type of herpes infection is usually caused by *herpes simplex virus type 1*, and is most often spread from mouth to mouth (and often from parent to child). Genital herpes is usually caused by *herpes simplex virus type 2*. However, there is no hard and fast rule about this. While type 1 likes the mouth best and type 2 likes the genitals best, the virus can be transmitted from a site on one person's body to another site on the partner's body, depending on what body part contacts what. (If the virus is on the toe and if the toe spends a lot of time in someone else's ear, an infection in his or her ear can result.) The viral type does not change when the site of infection changes. If you received genital herpes from a type 1 herpes simplex cold sore on your partner, your genital herpes sores will still be type 1. There is no change of the virus type when it now appears on the genital skin. So your partner could have received herpes of the mouth from a parent at age three, have had no symptoms, and still have transmitted the virus to your genitals thirty years later!

So be careful before calling the divorce lawyer. Talk the problem out with your partner. Don't let herpes alone come between you. Be honest and demand honesty. Possibly your partner was with another partner and your genital herpes was the first sign—but possibly not. An honest discussion about herpes may even bring you closer together.

Herpes of the newborn is a deforming, blinding, often fatal disease. Should I give up my plans to have children?

No. Since herpes is spread from active skin infection and not from latent infection, a newborn baby can be infected with herpes only if he or she is born while the virus is active. *Neonatal herpes* generally occurs if the baby's skin becomes infected during the birth process. If herpes is latent in the mother, there is no virus along the birth canal to infect the baby. If herpes sores are present at the time of labor, then (and only then) a cesarean section may be required to reduce the possibility of direct contact between the infection and the baby. Before birth, the membranes surrounding the baby are a natural barrier that helps to prevent the virus from travelling from the mother's skin to the baby's skin. If the membranes rupture (the bag of water breaks) and a herpes sore on or near the vagina is active, a cesarean section is often performed as an emergency operation. If no sores are present, however, normal labor may safely proceed. Many centers are now studying the use of regular oral acyclovir during the last two to four weeks of pregnancy to prevent reactivations and allow for a normal vaginal delivery. You may wish to discuss this with your doctor.

In order to avoid giving herpes to your baby, you must also tell your doctor that you have herpes (or that a previous partner had or your present partner has herpes). During labor, the doctor will carefully inspect your genitals, especially the external genital area, for herpes sores. You must take an active role and discuss the problem well in advance with your doctor. Regular, careful examinations of the external genitals by your physician during the last two or three weeks of pregnancy may be useful, depending upon how frequently you get recurrences. You and the doctor should increase your awareness of your herpes outbreaks—what they feel like, what they look like, and so on. If possible, your doctor will take a herpes culture from the skin around the vagina during labor; in the unlikely event that a sore has been missed, there will be time to watch and treat the baby, if necessary. The chances that a mother with recurrent genital herpes will give birth to a baby who becomes ill with neonatal herpes are only about one in several thousands, as long as you and your doctor are aware of the status of your infection and are attuned to prevention.

A fetus can also get a herpes infection *inside* the womb. In this situation, herpes could have a harmful effect on the fetus before birth. This syndrome of *congenital herpes* is very rare. Some physicians believe that *primary herpes* (the first episode of herpes) in the mother may lead to infection in the womb, especially if primary herpes occurs in early pregnancy. However, the overwhelming majority of women who have primary herpes during the first two trimesters of pregnancy give birth to perfectly normal babies. Primary herpes in early pregnancy is not considered an absolute indication for abortion, although some women in this situation may choose to have abortions. One study from Seattle showed that one in five such situations (true primary herpes in the first trimester of pregnancy) led to a miscarriage where the fetus was shown to have been affected by herpes in the uterus. Because this situation is so uncommon, the study may have underestimated or overestimated the true incidence. Follow-up unpublished studies from the same medical center suggest that one in five may be an overestimate. Nothing specific can be done to prevent congenital herpes, but the risk is very low. In fact, even women with a proven herpes infection inside the womb often have completely normal and unaffected babies. Most healthy and well-nourished babies who are born to women with herpes are very unlikely to develop problems.

When you consider how many new mothers have had a genital herpes infection, it may seem surprising that herpes of the newborn remains an uncommon disease. Some physicians believe that antibodies account for this low incidence. Most people with herpes make plenty of herpes antibodies—proteins that neutralize the virus on contact (see chapter 2). The antibodies probably get into the amniotic fluid in which the baby floats, coating the baby in a layer of protection. Antibodies may knock out the virus before (or after) it gets onto the baby's skin. The exact role of protective antibodies is not fully known. However, we do know that compared with recurrent genital herpes in the mother, primary genital herpes during late pregnancy (where antibodies are not yet available) results in a much greater risk to the newborn baby. Neonatal herpes is very uncommon, while recurrent genital herpes in pregnancy is extremely common.

Recent studies by Charles Prober and Ann Arvin at Stanford University have focused on primary infection as a risk for neonatal herpes. They have looked specifically at women in the third trimester of their pregnancy who do not have any antibodies to herpes and who are susceptible to primary type 2 genital herpes because their partners have type 2 genital herpes. This "discordance of pairs" is a specific situation in which a pregnant woman could be expected to develop a primary infection. The data show that women with true primary infections are at much greater risk of transmitting their infection to their babies than are women with recurrent infections.

Another way to look at this is that if a pregnant woman knows she has herpes and has had it for awhile, she is protected by nature from transmitting herpes to the newborn in most cases. Her baby acquires immunity to herpes from her. If she sheds virus asymptomatically, her baby will probably be exposed, if at all, to only a small amount of virus, which will probably be readily neutralized by her immunity. If, on the other hand, the baby is exposed to a primary infection, a large amount of virus is present, often on the cervix, and the pregnant woman has not yet developed protective antibodies. That is the really dangerous situation. Recurrent herpes in the pregnant woman, which is more common, is usually less problematic. In fact, some epidemiologists feel that there is a significantly greater threat to the mother from having a cesarean than there is to the infant who might be exposed to a recurrent lesion. This is still controversial, but it does point to the fact that part of the problem with herpes in pregnancy is the number of unnecessary cesareans performed. There are exceptions to everything, of course, but it is OK to get pregnant and have a baby even though you or your partner have herpes. If you are pregnant and your sexual partner has herpes and you don't, then you should be very careful. Follow all safe sexual practices during the first two trimesters and especially during the third trimester. In fact, it is safest in this situation to avoid sexual contact during the third trimester. Do not avoid getting pregnant because of herpes, but do take time to understand the issues.

Can herpes cause cancer?

Does herpes infection lead to cancer? Several years ago, investigators noticed that people with more active sex lives had a statistically higher chance of getting cancer of the cervix. Celibacy, then, is one way to avoid cervical cancer. In fact, this cancer almost never occurs in Catholic nuns. There is no question that sex causes cervical cancer. Herpes antibodies are much more likely to be present in blood samples from women with cervical cancer than in blood samples from women without this cancer. Does this prove that herpes caused the cancer—or does it only show that herpes relates to sexual activity and that something else about sexual activity relates to cervical cancer? Herpes does not seem to cause cervical cancer. Human papillomavirus, which causes genital warts, is now receiving the most attention in research into cervical cancer. Certain subtypes of this virus appear to be the main causes of cervical cancer. As the evidence mounts for papillomavirus as a cause, the association between herpes and cervical cancer is rapidly diminishing.

Regardless of the possible causes of cervical cancer, every woman can take steps to prevent complications of this easily detected cancer. Happily, cervical cancer grows very slowly at first and is easy to detect in its early stages. Cure is virtually guaranteed if cervical cancer is detected early. Major surgery is generally not required to halt the disease in the early stages. Easy detection is accomplished by the *Papanicolaou (Pap) smear*. I recommend that women with herpes have annual Pap smears—not only as a precaution but also for peace of mind. The Pap test is a quick, simple, and painless test that samples the coating on the cervix (the mouth of the womb). Under the microscope, cancer cells in the specimen can be detected in their earliest stage. All women should have this test done regularly, and women who have had herpes or any sexually transmitted disease should have it done at least once a year. Beyond a regular Pap test, no other precautions against cervical cancer are necessary.

Conclusion

Herpes is able to cause a recurrent skin infection. People most often remain totally unaware that they have this infection. However, once herpes has been diagnosed, its recurrence can usually be clearly recognized. Avoiding transmission comes naturally once you understand the active phases of infection and begin to use safer sex practices. Control of your infection comes gradually as your own army of immunity takes over and fights off each recurrence with efficient killing power. With time, the frequency of recurrences may diminish. The virus may cause a terrible infection in some newborn babies, but this syndrome tends to occur most commonly where the mother is experiencing her first-ever (primary) genital infection. Mothers with recurrent genital herpes are largely protected from this complication by their own immunity, which is passed on to the child more efficiently than the virus itself. Neonatal herpes is a highly preventable and uncommon disease, and it is almost always under the control of the mother and her physician if she knows she has herpes and discusses the problem.

Cervical cancer, which is probably caused by human papillomavirus, is statistically associated with herpes as well. It is highly doubtful that herpes actually causes this cancer. Through the yearly Pap smear, this cancer can be easily detected and effectively dealt with. It is unlikely to occur, herpes or no herpes.

Is herpes an incurable disease that kills babies and causes cervical cancer? No. On the contrary, herpes is an extremely common virus infection, poorly understood by many people and further sensationalized by the media. It is a nuisance, without doubt. It can be a problem when it recurs very frequently. Safe and effective drug therapy that reduces the frequency of both symptomatic and asymptomatic recurrences is now available. Herpes can sometimes result in serious complications, but people who have herpes can easily prevent these complications. If you have the right information, herpes is a syndrome that can be under your control.

2
Herpes Simplex: The Virus

*We live in a dancing matrix of viruses; they dart, rather
like bees, from organism to organism... passing around
heredity as though at a great party... If this is true, the
odd virus disease, on which we must focus so much
of our attention in medicine, may be looked on
as an accident, something dropped.*

−LEWIS THOMAS
*The Lives of a Cell:
Notes of a Biology Watcher*

A short history of herpes

Herpes infections are not new. Over twenty-five centuries ago
Hippocrates, the father of medicine, coined the word "herpes"
from the Greek "to creep." Medicine in his time was descriptive;
diseases were classified according to their appearance. The diseases that Hippocrates called herpes are now known to be several
different skin maladies with several different names and causes.

In the first part of this century, scientists discovered the "filter-
able virus," a particle so small that it could pass through a paper
filter and could not be seen with the microscope and yet was fully
capable of causing infection. It was not long before microbiologists
had identified many different viruses capable of causing different
diseases. Some examples are polio, hepatitis, influenza, and rhi-
novirus (the common cold). The virus that causes herpes was
identified as herpes simplex. The cause of herpes infections
became further understood and the different kinds of herpes viruses further classified.

A great step forward in understanding viruses was the development of the technology for growing viruses outside the body—i.e.,
in vitro (in the test tube). Since viruses are parasites of cells,

they need cells in which to grow. The first advance in the field was the discovery that human cells could be stimulated to grow artificially by giving them the right nutrients and keeping them at the right temperature. Cells are the "unit system" of the body. They contain all the parts necessary for reproduction and metabolism; that is, they can make new copies of themselves and carry out the chemical processes needed for life. Furthermore, each type of cell in the body has a special function. It might specialize in moving body parts (muscle cells), building structures (bone cells), filtering out poison (kidney cells), detoxifying poison (liver cells), guarding the body surface (epithelial cells), killing foreign invaders (lymphocytes and leukocytes), or carrying oxygen to other cells (erythrocytes).

Pick any organ or system of the body—whether it be for pumping blood or for thinking. If you look at a slice of this tissue under the microscope, you will see different cells, each doing its thing. Figure 1 is from such a slice of normal skin. The cells can be seen lined up according to function. The epithelial cells are the special targets of the herpes simplex virus. Note the thick layer of keratin, a waxy outer coating of skin that forms a natural physical barrier to ward off invasion by infection.

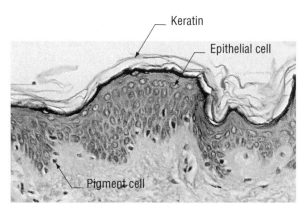

Figure 1: A microscope view of a slice of skin. As long as the waxy outer coating of keratin stays unbroken, it helps to prevent herpes simplex virus from finding its target— the epithelial (skin) cells. The cells with the dark pigment (called melanin) give the skin its color.

Viruses are grown in the laboratory by allowing them to infect normal body cells growing in the test tube. First the body cells must be grown in culture. To do this, a piece of tissue is placed in a test tube with chemicals and enzymes and carefully chopped up. The separated cells are then given nutrients like sugar, amino acids, and vitamins. If everything goes well, the cells will soon grow and multiply. Figure 2 shows skin cells grown in culture. No longer specialized for skin, these cells are all of the same type, called fibroblasts.

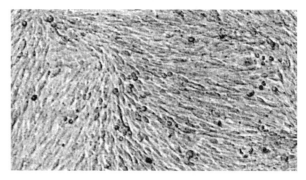

Figure 2: A microscopic view of human fibroblast cells grown in tissue culture. Cells in the laboratory look like this if they are healthy—not affected by a virus or anything else. Different viruses can be detected by the changes they induce in these cells.

Once scientists were able to grow cells in vitro (outside the body), getting viruses to grow inside those cells became easier. Viruses were soon purified, analyzed, and classified. Herpes simplex virus could be detected from sores, on the genitals and elsewhere. At first, herpes was not considered to be a sexually transmitted disease. It was later shown, however, that the greater the number of sexual partners an individual had, the greater the risk of contracting herpes.

By the late 1960s, herpes of the newborn had been linked to an active herpes infection in the mother at the time of birth. This marked the beginning of an explosive period of herpes research.

Cervical cancer was (erroneously) connected with herpes. As more became known about herpes, it became more widely publicized, and the public alarm made good press. More people with bothersome sores sought medical help. At the same time, the population became more sexually active. Society loosened many sexual taboos. Casual sexual contact and oral sex became more frequent. Possibly the most important factor in increasing herpes, however, was the change of birth control methods. As people left behind condoms and foam for the convenience of the IUD and the pill, they left behind effective barriers to infection.

Today, we have a reservoir of virus in the community that is so large that herpes has become almost unavoidable. Today, ten times as many people seek help from a physician for genital herpes as they did twenty years ago. Studies in Vancouver, British Columbia, show that 20 percent of women who have ever had sex have genital herpes type 2. Once they have had six or more sexual partners, about 40 percent of women have genital herpes. Having had more than ten sexual partners gives women a risk of almost 60 percent for genital herpes. Studies in African-American populations show that men have an incidence of about 40 percent and women an incidence of about 60 percent. In all studies and all populations, men have a slightly lower risk of acquiring genital herpes. Their different anatomy seems to make them slightly less likely to get herpes from a partner. Yet both sexes are at significantly high risk—a risk that is not related to their exposure to partners who are known to have herpes. Consistent use of safer sex practice will lower the risks, but unfortunately, most couples do not use them. You don't have to be a statistician to see the problem we face now and in the future.

What is a virus, anyway?

A virus is a very small living thing. It is so small that it can pass through something as fine as a coffee filter. It cannot live on its own. A virus contains either DNA or RNA (hereditary material that passes on characteristics to the next generation of viruses). As depicted in the graphic illustration (see plate 1, page 95), this hereditary material is surrounded by a protective coat made of protein and sometimes by another protective outer coat called an *envelope,* which is made of fatty and protein-like material. An electron micrograph of herpes is shown in figure 3.

A virus lives according to all known laws of heredity and natural selection. Its biological job is to make copies of itself, called *daughter particles.* A virus reproduces in a straightforward fashion. First, since it is a parasite, it seeks a host cell that provides a suitable environment. Each virus has its own favorite type of host cell. Which cell the virus likes best partly determines which disease it causes. For example, hepatitis viruses like liver cells, while herpes simplex viruses like skin and nerve cells.

Plate 2 shows how herpes infects an epithelial (skin) cell (see plate 2, page 96, simplified for clarity). After finding the cell, the virus attaches itself (probably to special receptors or receiving sites) to the outer layer of the cell, called the *membrane.* It then "undresses" itself and injects its hereditary material (DNA) into the cell. The DNA finds its way to the cell nucleus, where it uses the cell's own machinery to make virus daughter particles. Usually this reproduction of new viruses stops the host cell from living for itself. After new virus particles are made, the human cell bursts and dies, scattering daughter particles around to neighboring cells, where the cycle is repeated.

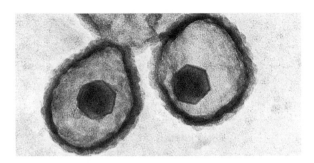

Figure 3: An electron micrograph of two herpes simplex viruses. Note the highly organized geometric shape of the nucleocapsid surrounded by a large, shapeless envelope.

Viruses have a different relationship with human cells than bacteria do. Bacteria are self-sufficient—living all on their own. A virus is a parasite; it survives by taking over the host cell machinery. That is why a virus is so hard to kill. Bacteria (gonorrhea, for example) don't need a host cell in which to live and grow. They are a part of the plant kingdom in nature and need only basic nutrients (carbohydrates, proteins, and so forth). Because bacteria can make so many of their own products, they are easy to kill with antibiotics (such as penicillin), which interrupt some manufacturing process that is vital to the bacteria but is of no concern to the human body. (Penicillin, for example, interrupts the manufacture of the bacterial cell wall. It has no effect on human cells, because animal cells do not have a cell wall.) The virus needs its host cell, however, and since the virus uses the host cell's manufacturing system for its own life cycle, many chemicals that kill the virus also interrupt the normal host metabolism. That is why, to date, there is no cure for the common cold and no cure for herpes.

We are learning more and more about viruses, however. As researchers find things that viruses do that are unique to the virus, so are they able to find ways of killing the virus without harming the host. In fact, researchers can now use the special chemistry of herpes viruses to select and kill cancer cells. This is done by transferring parts of viral DNA to a cancerous tumor, using another virus as a vector, or carrier.

What stops a viral infection?

The growth cycle of a virus is eventually halted by the coordinated strategy of the body's immune system, which has two major components: the *humoral* system and *cell-mediated* system (see plate 15, page 102). The humoral system uses cells called lymphocytes to recognize viral glycoproteins. When triggered by these glycoproteins, the B lymphocytes produce proteins called antibodies. The antibodies cling to the virus particles and inactivate them. The cell-mediated component of the immune system uses fighter cells called T lymphocytes. T lymphocytes called CD8 cells (also called "cytotoxic" T cells) look around for infected cells that contain viral proteins to which they have been sensitized. When they find such a cell, they attack and kill it. CD4 cells (also called "helper" T cells) help by stimulating T cells and B cells to grow and do their jobs. CD4 cells are the main target of HIV, and their deple-tion causes many of the problems in AIDS patients whose cell-mediated immunity is depleted.

Macrophages (see plate 5, page 97) then come along as janitors and clean up the mess, leaving room for healthy, unaffected cells to grow and replace the old.

Why don't we develop immunity to herpes? (The story of latent infection)

We really do develop immunity to herpes. The body's immune sys-tem is very effective at stopping a recurrence once it starts. But how, then, is it able to start at all? Herpes simplex has two tricks up its sleeve to beat the system. Although most of the virus is wiped out by the body's defenses, some virus finds its way up the nerve endings that give feeling to the affected areas of skin.

The body's sensory nervous network gives physical sensations such as pain, temperature sensation, and touch sensation. To accomplish this, nerve fibers extend to all areas of skin like a branching network of phone cables supplying many houses with phone service. Groups of nerve fibers gather up the electrical input from several areas into one cable for transmission to the brain and feed into their local switching station, called a *ganglion*. The ganglia lie next to the spinal cord—the main cable—and house the cell machinery for all the nerve fibers. There are sever-al ganglia running along the spinal cord from top to bottom.

The herpes virus wastes no time in establishing its latent state, penetrating the nerve fiber (axon) very quickly after infecting the skin cell. The nucleocapsid (containing the DNA) travels up the nerve fiber and stops when it gets to the ganglion, shown in figure 4. In some of the nerve cells, the virus comes to rest; in others it proceeds with its active growth cycle. Herpes decides very quick-ly whether it will cause a latent or an active infection in each cell it infects. Why does it go to rest in some cells (*latent infection*) while growing actively (*productive infection*) in others? A dual infection system (latent and productive) gives the virus a strong persistence mechanism. Within the nerve cells identified for latent (dormant) infection, there appears to be no significant damage to the nerve. In fact, this infection state is so quiet that the body's defenses do not even sense a problem. While the body's immune system effectively eradicates active viral infection in the skin, it does not even try to put up a fight against latent infection in the nerve. Herpes is so effective at establishing itself in the latent state that, in laboratory tests, it seems to be able to become latent even if a genetic mutation prevents the virus from normal reproduction.

Figure 4: During active skin infection, while the infected epithelial cells are going through their battle with the immune system, it is thought that the nerve fibers that supply sensation to the affected areas of skin also become infected (lower box). The virus travels up the nerve fiber until it gets to the core of the cell inside the ganglion. There it stops. Unlike the productive and explosive infection occuring on the skin, infection of the nerve cell results in quiet, or latent, infection that persists (upper box).

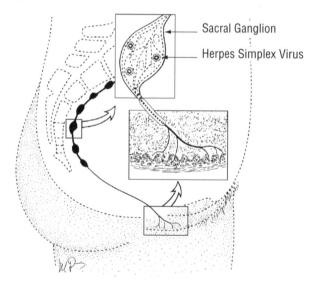

Sacral Ganglion

Herpes Simplex Virus

Several copies of the viral DNA are present inside each latently infected human nerve cell. It is not known whether this occurs because several virus particles attack a single cell or because one virus particle produces several latent copies of itself. Many nerve cells in an affected ganglion may be infected. The viral DNA exists inside the neuron in the form of circles that are extrachromosomal (not incorporated into the human host cell's DNA). This viral DNA is associated with cellular proteins called histones. From its latent state, virus can be cultivated from ganglion cells removed in autopsies, under very special conditions of care, called *cocultivation*. In the body, reactivation from latent to productive infection occurs from time to time. Reactivation can be induced by a neurosurgeon operating near a latently infected ganglion. In such a case, herpes recurs at the original skin site as a postoperative complication.

Inside the neuronal nucleus, herpes simplex virus makes a type of RNA known as a *latency-associated transcript*, or LAT. LATs are not actually required to ensure that latency occurs, although they do seem to make it easier for herpes to reactivate. Only some of the factors that determine latency of herpes simplex virus come from the virus, however. Many other factors that govern herpes simplex viral latency in neurons are controlled strictly by certain characteristics of the host nerve cell.

Every ganglion is different, and every person is different. On the face, type 1 herpes simplex virus tends to recur more than type 2 herpes simplex virus, because type 1 reactivates more efficiently from the trigeminal ganglia located near the brain stem. On the genitals and buttocks, type 2 tends to recur more than type 1, because type 2 reactivates more efficiently from the sacral ganglia, located near the base of the spine (figure 4). A strain of virus that reactivates infrequently in one person may reactivate frequently in another. Viral factors are important, such as the virulence of the specific viral strain, the quantity of virus infecting the person, the viral type (type 1 versus type 2) and other genetic factors of the virus and its heritage. Human host factors include the susceptibility of the infected person as determined by heredity and immunity, whether or not there has been previous exposure to another strain of herpes simplex virus, and the length of exposure to the virus. Latent virus remains dormant holding the potential to reactivate when triggered to do so.

Latency: the reactivation process from sacral ganglia to genital skin

Herpes simplex virus follows a defined route upon reactivation. It travels down the nerve fibers that emanate from the specific nerve cell that is reactivating. The cells harboring latent virus are logically in the ganglia where nerve fibers lead from the genital skin. In general, then, herpes travels back down nerve fibers in the same general vicinity as those first affected. After travelling back down to the end of the nerve fiber, the virus reaches the surface of a new, uninfected skin cell, attaches itself to receptors at the cell surface, and penetrates the healthy skin cell. Since nerve fibers tend to branch into related groups of smaller fibers, herpes often appears on the skin as a cluster of tiny sores, each representing the result of one virus particle recurring at one cell at the end of one tiny nerve fiber. Then, the active state begins again and a new recurrent infection takes place. The recurrent infection once again signals danger to the body's immune system, and the antibodies and cells go to work halting the active infection. Recurrences are often less severe than first-time skin infection, because neutralizing antibodies were made the first time. T lymphocytes were targeted and are already there, waiting to attack emerging *virions* (daughter virus particles). At the time of the first infection, if the first infection was truly primary, antibodies had not yet formed, and so lesions took longer to heal, affected more skin, and caused more blisters and symptoms. Now the immune system is able to halt the recurrence in short order. However, preventing the reactivation from beginning is not so easy, because the virus hibernates in a quiet or latent state in a nerve cell and then travels back to the skin via the inside of the nerve's fiber until the reactivation process has begun, thus sneaking by the body's immune system until the reactivation process has already been set in motion.

Remember, herpes has *two* tricks. The first is its ability to remain latent in the nerve cells. The second is its ability to go from one cell to another without ever leaving the cell environment. Suppose you decided to rob houses in your neighborhood by going from your house to your neighbor's house without ever going outdoors. In that way you could avoid the police. To go a step further, you could send a signal to a carpenter in your neighbor's house telling him or her to build a self-enclosed bridge to your house. This is exactly what herpes simplex virus does. The cell with virus fuses with its neighbor cell by inducing bridges. So many cells may fuse that a *multinucleated giant cell* is formed. (These giant cells are so specific for herpes that they are one way the virologist can tell if a virus culture is growing herpes.)

Why is this bridging important? With most viruses, immunity is a sufficient defense to prevent a recurrence. The basis for preventive vaccines like polio and measles is that the vaccine stimulates antibody production: when the virus comes along, it is neutralized by the antibodies before it spawns a disease. Since antibody is a very good virus poison, and since most viruses grow inside cells and then release themselves into the interstitial (extracellular) environment when the cell bursts, disease cannot recur. Antibodies are waiting, and the infection is nipped in the bud. Herpes is different. Most herpes-infected cells do burst, and most of the herpes virus is neutralized, but antibodies cannot easily travel to the inside of a cell to attack a virus—and herpes is busy building bridges *before* its growth has progressed to the cell-bursting stage. A few virions saunter happily to a neighboring cell, safely protected inside the cell. Other emerging young virions that break outside to the interstitial spaces will be killed effectively and quickly by neutralizing antibodies, but a select few stay inside cells and live on for a short time to infect healthy neighboring cells. Quite a trick! Of course, the immune system cuts this process off by using its lymphocytes and macrophages to identify infected cells and clear up the mess—just as our imaginary scheme for robbing houses would not get very far before the police put a stop to it.

Antibodies are very helpful in limiting the severity of herpes recurrences, but the immune system cannot prevent recurrences from reactivating entirely. Recent clinical studies with one of the new vaccine candidates (Chiron-Biocine) have, in fact, shown that boosting the immune system with that herpes vaccine does not reduce recurrence rates or prevent infections in partners. Vaccines may very well induce many kinds of immunity, including neutralizing antibodies and viral-specific immune cells. We know that the immune system naturally and effectively controls the severity of herpes infections. However, despite the best fight the immune system can muster, recurrences of herpes may reactivate as small sores before the body reacts to shut down the process.

Herpes is very effective at hiding from its enemies. Hippocrates chose a remarkably apt name for herpes—to creep.

What is a herpes virus?

The herpes family of viruses includes eight different viruses that affect human beings. The official names are known by numerical designation as *human herpes virus* 1 through 8 (HHV1-HHV8):

1. **Human herpes virus 1 (HHVI)** is the official name for *herpes simplex virus type 1*, discussed at length in this book. It can cause cold sores or herpes of the eye, and it commonly causes first episodes of genital herpes.

2. **Human herpes virus 2 (HHV2)** is the official name for *herpes simplex virus type 2*, the most common cause of genital herpes and, less frequently, herpes of the newborn. It is much less commonly associated with facial and eye infections.

3. **Human herpes virus 3 (HHV3)** is the official name for *herpes zoster virus* (also called *varicella zoster virus*), the cause of chickenpox. Like its close relative, herpes simplex virus, herpes zoster likes to infect skin cells and nerve cells. The first three human herpes viruses are called *neurotropic* (also called "*alpha*") because of their characteristic love for nerve cells. Chickenpox is the primary (first-time) infection with herpes zoster. This virus may also recur along nerve fiber pathways, causing multiple sores where nerve fibers end on skin cells. Because the entire ganglion tends to reactivate with this virus, the physical severity of a recurrence is generally much worse than a recurrence of herpes simplex virus. Recurrent varicella virus infection of the skin is commonly known as either *zoster* or *shingles*. Both words translate from different languages into "belt" which describes the pattern in which the lesions appear on the body. Shingles only occurs once (or, rarely, twice). If you are told that your frequently recurrent herpes infection is frequent herpes zoster or shingles infection, a misdiagnosis has probably been made; have this checked out carefully with a reliable virus test.

4. **Human herpes virus 4 (HHV4)** is the official name of *Epstein-Barr virus*, the major cause of infectious mononucleosis, or mono ("kissing disease").

5. **Human herpes virus 5 (HHV5)** is the official name of *cytomegalovirus* (CMV). CMV is also a cause of mono. It can be sexually transmitted, can cause problems to newborns, and can cause hepatitis. Occasionally it is transmitted by blood transfusion. It is very common among homosexual men and is often associated with (but is not the cause of) AIDS. CMV infection is one of the most difficult complications of AIDS, often leading to severe visual problems or even blindness, infection of the gastrointestinal tract, diarrhea, and a variety of other difficult problems—even death. For a virus that barely causes a problem in most people with normal immunity, it can be amazingly nasty in people with severely compromised immunity.

6. **Human herpes virus 6 (HHV6)** is a recently observed agent found in the blood cells of a few patients with a variety of diseases. It is known to be the cause of roseola in small children and can also cause a variety of other illnesses associated with fever in that age group, even where the typical roseola rash is missing. This infection apparently accounts for many of the cases of convulsions associated with fever in infancy (*febrile seizures*).

7. **Human herpes virus 7 (HHV7)** is even more recently observed. Like all human herpes viruses, HHV6 and 7 are ubiquitous. In other words, they are so common that most of humankind has been infected at some point—usually early in life. It is not at all clear what clinical effects this virus causes.

8. **Human herpes virus 8 (HHV8)** was recently discovered in the tumors called *Kaposi's Sarcoma* (KS) that are found in people with AIDS (and are otherwise very rare). KS forms purplish tumors in the skin and other tissues of some people with AIDS and has been very difficult to treat with medication. HHV8 may also cause other cancers, including certain lymphomas associated with AIDS. The fact that these cancers are caused by a

virus may explain why such complications tend to occur in people with AIDS when their immune systems begin to fail. The discovery also provides new hope that specific treatments for these tumors will be developed that target the virus.

3
Genital Herpes:
The Symptoms

Yes, it is the exact location of the soul that I am after.
The smell of it is in my nostrils. I have caught glimpses of it
in the body diseased. If only I could tell it. Is there no
mathematical equation that can guide me? So much
pain and pus equals so much truth?

—RICHARD SELZER
Mortal Lessons: Notes on
the Art of Surgery

What are the symptoms of genital herpes?

Herpes, like any other infection, causes a spectrum of symptoms
from very mild to very severe. There are people whose lab tests
prove they have had infection but who show no symptoms whatsoever, while, on the other hand, there are people whose symptoms are so severe that they result in extreme disability or even
death. An example of the latter would be a newborn baby who
became infected with herpes that disseminated throughout the
body.

When it causes infection in a normal person, however, genital
herpes almost never results in severe disability or death. Most
people with genital herpes are at the opposite end of the spectrum. They have been exposed to genital herpes and have developed latent infection and antibodies but have never had any
symptoms of active infection. It is difficult, then, to paint a single
picture of what herpes infection is like. The symptoms depend not
only on the severity of infection but also on its site, which in turn
is largely determined by the site of inoculation. In other words,
where did the herpes virus find its easiest access to epithelial cells
of the skin? For the most part, herpes simplex prefers mucous

membranes, where the skin is thin. These include areas like the labia (lips) of the vagina and the lips of the mouth. However, any area of the body may be fair territory for herpes. If a finger has a tiny crack on it (which it commonly does), any herpes simplex virus sitting on the finger can easily find its way to an epithelial cell. In general, though, it is difficult for the virus to enter the skin on the hand and other thick-skinned areas. However, any time there is excessive moisture, and especially if there is trauma or injury that compromises the normal protection of the area, the setting is ideal for herpes to be transmitted. (For further information on autoinoculation, see chapter 5.)

First episodes of genital herpes can be classified in three categories: *primary infection, nonprimary initial infection,* and *recurrent infection.*

Primary infection

The person who experiences a true primary infection has never previously been exposed to any herpes simplex virus. Before infection there is no history of cold sores, there is no history of exposure to cold sores, and no immunity to herpes has ever developed. The absence of specific immunity is crucial, because it allows for easier infection. The body, in its defense against its first attack by herpes, makes antibodies that can neutralize the herpes virus quite effectively. Also, immune cells of the body learn how to target and destroy the virus. As a result, once specific immune cells and antibodies are present, herpes infections are usually much milder.

The first infection is called a primary infection if no previous antibody to either type 1 or type 2 herpes simplex virus is present. It is only possible to know for sure that a person does not have such antibodies by performing a special blood test. Many people with antibodies to either type 1 or type 2 herpes simplex virus have no recollection of cold sores, genital herpes, or any other symptom related to herpes. During a true primary infection, the virus can be inoculated, or transferred, to surrounding areas of skin. Infection may be much more severe because no immunity specific to herpes is yet present. More sores will usually develop during a true primary, especially in women. The person may feel generally sick, usually with a flu-like illness that feels very much like any other viral infection, causing muscle aches and pains and possibly fever and headaches. Primary infection causes a spectrum of disease symptoms, however. For most people, primary infection will actually pass entirely unnoticed or will cause symptoms or signs that are atypical and may be readily misdiagnosed. An atypical primary infection, for example, could produce only a small amount of vaginal discharge, some difficulty with getting urination started, leg pains, headaches, or vaginitis of unknown cause. A woman may only find out she is in the midst of a primary infection when a routine Pap smear comes back showing active cervical herpes. In a recent case I saw, the family physician noted only some mild redness of the cervix.

When genital sores erupt, they usually do so at the site of inoculation, which is usually on the external genitals. Sores generally look like a cluster of small blisters filled with clear or whitish fluid. The classical herpes sore, seen in plate 8a, page 99, is just this: a group of small blisters (*vesicles*) on a red base of inflamed skin.

In many cases, these blisters are never seen, and the first signs of infection are small erosions of the skin called *ulcers*. Ulcers also tend to come in clusters or groups. They may feel like chafing of the skin or some other nonspecific irritation.

In women, herpes sores or lesions are usually on the external genitals, most commonly on the labia (lips) of the vagina. Another common site is the area covered by pubic hair. In men, sores are usually on the foreskin or the shaft of the penis or in the pubic area, but the glans (tip of the penis) is also possible territory. More than one of these areas may be affected during primary herpes. Sores may vary in size from very small (one to two millimeters) to very large (one to two centimeters). Sores are usually quite superficial, with the infection on the outermost layer of the skin. During a symptomatic primary infection, the skin often becomes raw, painful, and itchy. There may be a lot of inflammation at this time, because the body is attacking the virus. This response is healthy but may lead to quite a bit of distress. If sores are present around the urethral meatus—the spot where urine exits—urination may be quite uncomfortable. There may be *external dysuria*: a stinging sensation when urine contacts the sores. Some people feel that they have trouble getting the urine stream started. Sores may also appear on the thighs, on the buttocks, or around the anus. There may also be sores in other areas, such as the mouth. If oral contact occurred with the same sores that infected your genitals, a mouth infection may result. Rare sites of infection are the fingers, the breasts, and the eyes.

Often the lymph nodes are swollen in the *inguinal*, or groin, region. This means that the immune system is fighting off the virus. Lymph nodes are those "glands" that the doctor often feels for in the neck when you have a cold. Similar glands are present throughout the body. Those in the groin (see figure 5) are the areas of lymph drainage from the genital area. With genital infection, the groin lymph nodes may become swollen and tender to the touch, since the lymph system is an important component of the body's immune system.

The cervix (the mouth of the womb) is infected about 80 to 90 percent of the time during primary infection. Except for vaginal discharge, cervical infection causes little in the way of symptoms. Occasionally, herpes sores can be seen on the cervix. During primary infection, there is usually some herpes virus on the cervix, even when sores are not present. Infection of the cervix with herpes may cause a runny vaginal discharge. Vaginal discharge could also be caused by another infection going on at the same time, such as trichomoniasis, yeast, or bacterial vaginosis. It is also important to remember that vaginal discharge may be perfectly normal. In fact, whether or not there is discharge, a physician or a specially trained paramedical person must examine you for other treatable infections that may have been transmitted at the same time as herpes.

Figure 5: Location of the inguinal lymph nodes. These "glands," or lymph nodes, may become swollen and/or tender during a bout of herpes. Swelling is most common during primary herpes but may occur with recurrent herpes also.

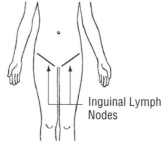

Inguinal Lymph Nodes

So, as you can see, primary herpes infections may cause anything from no symptoms to painful sores, sore throat, headache, and muscle pains, either alone or in combination. Symptoms will usually disappear within two to three weeks. The ulcer-like sores eventually scab over and the dry crusts fall off. This marks the end of the primary infection. Occasionally people find that they don't feel quite right for several weeks after their primary infection. There is no good explanation for this feeling.

Nonprimary initial infection

Not all first episodes of herpes are primaries, however. If a person having his or her first clinical experience with the virus is found to have blood test evidence of a previous exposure to type 1 herpes simplex virus, the episode is classified as a nonprimary initial infection. This person has an "immune memory" as a result of previous infection with herpes simplex type 1. More than 50 percent of people have some antibodies to type 1 herpes simplex virus, usually because they were exposed to someone's cold sores in childhood or because of a primary genital infection that gave no symptoms. So, in fact, the first clinical episode of genital herpes is usually not a true primary infection. Strengthening of the body's immune system by previous exposure makes nonprimary initial herpes very different from primary herpes. The antibodies and lymphocytes have already learned about type 1 herpes and are ready to be quickly activated when triggered by the presence of type 2 herpes. When infection occurs, the body combats the disease effectively and rapidly. The symptoms are essentially the same as for recurrent herpes. Recent studies suggest prove that type 1 herpes antibody partially protects against herpes type 2 infection, acting as a partial "vaccine." Over time, a person with preexisting immunity to herpes type 1 is theoretically less likely to pick up an infection with herpes type 2. However, previous type 1 antibody is clearly not totally protective against herpes type 2, since it is well known that people can acquire type 2 genital herpes after a lifelong history of type 1 (e.g., cold sores). In some studies, people with previous herpes simplex virus type 1 antibodies were almost three times less likely to pick up type 2 from an infected partner over time compared with people who had no previous type 1 herpes exposure. Even if a vaccine were to be only partially protective, though, it could still help, in theory, by raising the threshold of infection. Under such circumstances, it might require more virus, better inoculation, and better transmission circumstances for the body to take the new infection because of its underlying partial immunity. The partial immunity provided by type 1 antibody could thus provide a significant benefit by reducing the overall risk of acquiring type 2. This protection forms the basis of the studies of herpes vaccines currently under way; it has been the hope that vaccines may also provide significant clinical protection against infection. Results so far show that one of the vaccine candidates under study is not effective. Further studies continue with other candidate vaccines.

Recurrent infection

Like the typical nonprimary first episode, recurrent herpes is usually much milder than primary infection—again because of pre-existing immunity to herpes. Like the symptoms of a primary, the symptoms of recurrent herpes are the result of herpes infections of epithelial (skin) cells. However, recurrent infection results when virus travels back down the nerve pathway—often the same nerve fiber the virus originally traveled up on its way to causing latent infection of the ganglion (see figure 4) or a nerve branch from a close-by portion of the ganglion. When a recurrence takes place, however, the immune system is ready to deal with it.

Although the terms may be a bit confusing, we now know that many first episodes of genital herpes are actually recurrences. Even though it is the first clinically noticeable event, a special type-specific blood test (the Western blot) may show that a person is already immune to type 2 herpes simplex virus. This person may have had a primary or non-primary first episode in the past that went totally unnoticed (asymptomatic). Where a first episode is shown by this blood test to be recurrent, transmission may have taken place months or even years before the symptoms were noticed.

Of course, the vast majority of recurrent herpes infections are those that follow the first episode. We have learned, though, that the first episode may be a *primary* infection, a *non-primary* infection, or even a *recurrent* infection that was not previously recognized.

People with recurrent herpes are often troubled very little by physical ailments during recurrences. There are usually few sores. The sores, which may be single or multiple, tend to come in clusters, often grouped together on a small, reddened, inflamed base of skin. Recurrences of herpes go through a series of relatively predictable stages, all of which are described in detail in the next section of this chapter. Unlike primary infection, the recurrent herpes sequence usually takes just a few days from start to finish—an average of six days for men and five days for women. Compared with primary infection, recurrent lesions have less virus in them and are much less uncomfortable. Itchiness is very common. Recurrent sores are often tender to the touch, but they may not hurt a great deal if left alone. If, however, the sores are in a place where they are touched by urine or rubbed, pain may be more prominent. The general feeling of sickness that is usually present in the case of primary infection is now usually absent. Sores are in the same places as in primary herpes, except that the internal genitals and the cervix are much less often affected than in primary infection.

As with primary herpes, the symptoms of recurrent herpes depend on the area affected. Generally, one small area of one of the sites pictured in figure 6 is affected during one recurrence. Some people find that each recurrence is at precisely the same site. Others find that the site varies slightly each time. A sore may hurt when it occurs in one site but itch in another. Different recurrences may be of widely different severity, even in the same spot in the same person.

It is important to reiterate the wide range of severity here. Active recurrent herpes may be obvious when it comes in clusters of little blisters. But genital herpes may never be more severe than one very small sore on the labia or foreskin, around the anus, or on the thigh. It may be the size of a pencil eraser or as small as the sharpened lead point. The sore or chafing may never be painful at all and may not even itch. Herpes is variable and sometimes very atypical; it may hurt over here but itch over there. Assume that any break in the skin in an area depicted in figure 6 is herpes unless you know otherwise. Using a mirror, rub a wet finger lightly over the areas, looking for tender or red or swollen spots that might be active herpes. Get to know your herpes and anything else that is unusual on your genitals. You need to know if you're having a herpes outbreak when you're planning to have sex. If, much of the time, you have only minor skin problems or discomfort that only rarely turns into a classical herpes sore, then there could well be some other explanation for your sensations or skin breaks. For example, you might have a bacterial or yeast vaginal infection or you might be unsure about what is a sore and what is not. On the other hand, being too cavalier about genital discomfort is not good either. People commonly confuse herpes with other things, especially before they get to know their herpes. Herpes is often misidentified as a spider bite, especially on a leg or buttock or in an area remote from the genitals (see plate 9, page 100); a yeast infection (see plate 10, page 100); a hemorrhoid; pimples (on the buttocks, labia, etc.); shingles; water blisters; or cuts, slits, or chafing of the lips of the vagina caused by friction or soreness from vigorous contact.

The appearance and sequence of herpes sores are discussed in the coming pages. (For illustrations, refer to plates on pages 98 and 99.) The spectrum of variable severity must be kept in mind. The phases may all occur in the obvious sequence, or some phases may be skipped. They may last a week or an hour. Rarely, a person may need a hospital bed to recover from herpes. Someone in this situation will usually know the diagnosis! Others will never notice anything unusual. You can reach a happy medium of awareness of your body without overconcern about unrelated twinges. This happy medium may take a few months to achieve, but it will come. When herpes phases are inactive, virus is generally not on the skin, although exceptions to this occur from time to time in nearly all people with genital herpes. Avoiding transmission is relatively straightforward, although it requires a good understanding of the active phases of infection as well as of asymptomatic viral shedding and the susceptibility of the partner to infection. An active recurrence may never occur, or it may occur once in a lifetime,

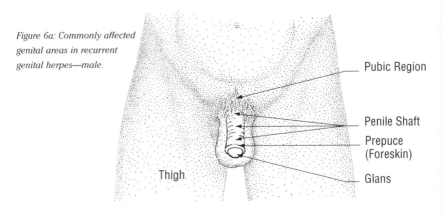

Figure 6a: Commonly affected genital areas in recurrent genital herpes—male.

Pubic Region

Penile Shaft

Prepuce (Foreskin)

Thigh

Glans

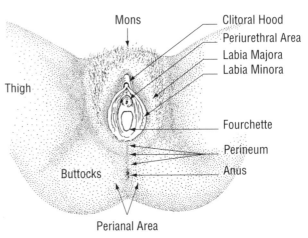

Figure 6b: Commonly affected genital areas in recurrent genital herpes—female.

Mons

Clitoral Hood

Periurethral Area

Labia Majora

Labia Minora

Thigh

Fourchette

Perineum

Anus

Buttocks

Perianal Area

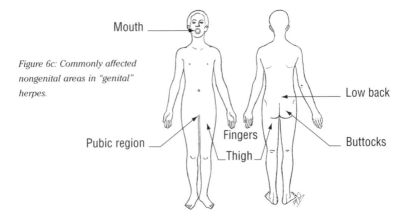

Mouth

Figure 6c: Commonly affected nongenital areas in "genital" herpes.

Low back

Pubic region

Fingers

Buttocks

Thigh

50

once in a year, or as often as three to four times a month. Type 2 herpes usually recurs at least a few times in the first year following infection. Although type 1 genital herpes can and does recur, the recurrences are about ten to fifteen times less frequent and are not so predictable.

What are the phases of herpes infections?

It is very important to know the phases, because living virus is very likely to be on the skin during the active phases. The phases of infection can be categorized as asymptomatic, prodrome (warning), early redness, edema, vesicles, wet ulcers, crusts, and healed.

During the *asymptomatic* phase, the virus is generally latent. Living in the ganglion, herpes is usually not on the skin. If you know what herpes feels and looks like and you've looked and found none, you can be confident that the risk of transmission at that specific time is far lower than during one of the active phases of infection. Herpes is only passed on when it is active on the skin. You can do a great deal to prevent transmission. However, there is a small risk that the virus may be reactivating even though your body does not sense an outbreak. Overall, asymptomatic shedding seems to occur on about 1 to 4 percent of days, depending on the patient population and the study. Safer sex consistently practiced during asymptomatic periods is the best way to reduce transmission risks. Suppressive, twice-daily antiviral medication substantially (but not completely) reduces the frequency of asymptomatic shedding. (These issues are discussed again at some length in subsequent chapters.)

Most (but not all) people with recurrences of herpes have a *prodrome,* or warning, that signifies that the virus has been reactivated and is on its way to the skin. As the virus activates, the nerve may react and symptoms may develop. The warning is different for different people. Recurrences often begin with some sensation or warning sign that something is wrong—for example, a pain in the leg or tingling or itching in one area of the genitals. Warning signs, if present, may occur for a few minutes or a few days. If there is a warning sign, it typically develops at the site of the future sore for a few hours before the outbreak begins. It may be a sensation such as localized burning, itching, tingling, or vague discomfort. The most common prodromal symptom is itching at the site before the lesions appear. Sometimes, though, warnings are not directly at the lesion site. Remember that nerves branch and that the virus reactivates very close to the body's central nervous system. Even though effectively eliminated by the immune system, herpes can irritate nerves at the ganglion or nerve site, rather than the skin site. For example, some people with herpes feel leg pains or buttock pains or sensations of burning on the side of the leg or bottom of one foot. Others develop a headache or a feeling like having a cold or the flu. Some people become emotionally irritable or down just before an outbreak. It may be something you've never noticed. It is useful to think about and identify your prodromal phase, if possible, because the prodromal phase tells you that the active sequence has started. At this time about 20 to 25 percent of people begin to have virus present on the skin. Skin contact with genital areas or other areas where you usually get sores should stop until the recurrence is completely over. It is very common for this phase to come and go without other phases following. After it is over, many people realize that they have had a warning, in the form of a vague sensation, below the level of consciousness, that something was amiss. Once a sore is there, there is the recognition, "Oh yeah, I felt that coming all day." Such recognition requires backtracking in your mind. If you have warnings, try to notice them as they occur, because they will help you to learn to recognize the active phase of infection early on. If you have no warnings, then your active phase of infection begins with the development of a lesion.

Next, *early redness* may be detected in a small area of skin (see plate 7a, page 98). It may feel itchy or painful to the touch or just sensitive. At this point, virus is beginning to grow inside the epithelial (skin) cells, and the immune system of antibodies and lymphocytes is being called back to work. The ensuing battle between defenses and virus causes inflammation or redness. Virus is in the skin, so contact with the area where a sore is developing is unwise. Sexual contact with the affected area—even protected sexual contact using safer sex practices—should not take place until the active phases of infection are over.

Soon, a sore begins to develop, beginning as a tiny spot of skin swelling or edema. The degree of swelling varies from one person to another and from one episode to another. Swelling is often so small that I hesitate to even mention this phase. For most people, the amount of skin edema is smaller in size than you might find from a tiny mosquito bite. This phase may be something that can be sensed as a swollen area, or it may be something that is felt by the fingers as one notices a bit of excess tissue at the site of tenderness. Sometimes, these areas of swelling may already have a small sore developing within the small area of swelling. Rarely, swelling from herpes can be very dramatic and result in a big swollen area. Herpes is often missed as the diagnosis in such cases, unless obvious sores are also present.

The next stage is *vesicles* (small blisters) (see plates 7b and 8a-d, pages 98 and 99). Vesicles are the small blisters filled with clear, whitish, or red (bloody) fluid that form on top of the early red or swollen patch. There may be only one vesicle, a few, or groups of so many that they run together. The tops of these blisters are very thin and come off easily, often oozing a little of the fluid. The fluid is the product of the sick, swollen skin cells that have been attacked by herpes. As the inflammation continues, itchiness and/or pain is often, but not always, present. Virus is virtually always present at this stage, so this is a good time to get a culture diagnosis. However, this stage is commonly skipped, especially in women with labial sores and men with sores under the foreskin, because these wet areas quickly macerate the blister and remove its top, leaving an ulcer underneath. In fact, just touching the vesicles may cause them to break and leak fluid. A vesicle poked with a cotton swab or the tip of your finger will be quite tender, even if it is not bothersome just sitting there. Avoid breaking vesicles on purpose, since there is nothing to be gained by doing this. Vesicles are usually grouped together on a red base of skin. They tend to form most obviously when herpes breaks out in an area where the skin is normally dry—for example, buttock, thigh, pubis, labia majora, or penile shaft.

Following the vesicle stage, lesions evolve into very superficial erosions, or *wet ulcers*, which are really the vesicles with their tops off (see plates 7c, 8e,f, pages 98 and 99). They glisten with wetness and may feel raw and/or tender to the touch. There may be one tiny sore that can be seen only with a magnifying lens, or there may a dozen large, tender ulcers. They may group together to form larger ulcers. Herpes ulcers are superficial; that is, they are right at the skin surface. They are not deep or ragged. They are generally somewhat round and wet. Tender to the touch is the rule, but there are exceptions. Virus is virtually always present at the base of the ulcer. Wet ulcers may look like a small cut or a red, swollen area. Slitlike (straight line) cuts that have absolutely no roundness to them in genital skin folds are often not caused by herpes. If that is all you experience, you should make certain that the sores you are getting are really herpes. Spread away the pubic hair, if necessary, for a good look, and use a magnifying mirror. Touch the sore with a cotton swab or a wet finger again to see if it is tender. This is really the area of the vesicle where the roof of the small blister has been removed. On areas of wet skin (labia minora, under the foreskin of the penis, clitoral hood, perineum, or perianal areas), sores may evolve so quickly that vesicles do not form.

Some people are not familiar or comfortable with identifying these areas as "sores" or "lesions" or "blisters" or "ulcers" because they are so mild in severity. Words like these may conjure up images for you that sound too severe. However, it is important to recognize symptoms, regardless of their severity, because doing so is what allows people who do not feel they have herpes to identify their herpes. Since virus may be present in either mild or painful sores, it is necessary to avoid the natural tendency to leave mild things unnoticed. I am not suggesting an obsession over normal or red spots on the skin. Herpes generally causes a specific sore of some type. The word "chafing" may ring more true for people whose recurrent sores are very mild. Areas of chafing are very superficial and often very small. They may be noticed only by their slight tenderness.

After the ulcer or chafing stage, the fluid in the ulcers begins to dry and some lesions may scab over with a *dry crust*, or scab (see plates 7e and 8h, pages 98 and 99). This phase marks the beginning of healing, and virus begins to disappear. The scab covers the raw ulcer just as a scab grows over a cut. At first the scab may be soft and wet and crumbly (see plates 7d and 8g, pages 98 and 99). If the scab is rubbed away, a wet ulcer remains underneath. As the sore dries, the crust hardens. Underneath, the skin grows anew. This is called re-epithelialization. While the crust is still there, virus may be present. Sexual contact with the area of the sore is still not advisable. The itch or pain may be leaving entirely, or the itch may just begin to worsen at this stage. The size of the lesion generally determines the size of the scab. Some small sores never have a crust stage and seem to melt away from ulcer to nothing. Others always form a dry crust. Scabbing is also very variable and tends to occur mainly on dry skin areas where lesions begin with the vesicle stage.

The sores are *healed* when the crust falls off or the lesion dries without forming a crust, completing the cycle of active infection (see plates 8i,j, page 99). Healing may leave a residual red mark, as a healed cut does. These spots may also be whitish rather than red, or they may in some other way look different from the unaffected skin. The marks may be slightly tender, but the surface is definitely healed with new skin that is smooth and knit back together and feels normal to the touch. The visible mark may last for weeks or for only a few days. Some people never get marks. Virus growth is over; only healing is active at this stage. Safer sexual (protected) contact with this area can now be resumed. In recurrent herpes, the healed phase generally occurs five to ten days after the appearance of the vesicle stage, although the time may be measured in hours or (rarely) in weeks. The "natural history" of a primary herpes outbreak is approximately three weeks. Not every phase occurs in every person. One or several of the phases may be skipped; for example, warnings may occur and no sores develop; ulcers may develop with no warning or blisters; or ulcers may heal with no crust stage. The stages are still important, however. When no symptoms are present and no sores are visible (and you've looked), or when only residual redness is left, the active infection is over and you are in the asymptomatic phase.

What are the trigger factors?

Several studies suggest that latent herpes may reactivate because of trigger factors. These factors are poorly understood, however, and are for the most part unavoidable. The known trigger factors include the menstrual cycle; emotional stress; another illness, especially with fever; sexual intercourse; surgery; injury; sunlight; and certain medications.

Each person's trigger factor is different. For example, while many women get herpes only during a certain part of the menstrual cycle, the trigger day of the cycle varies from woman to woman. One study suggested that more women develop recurrences five to twelve days before the onset of their next menstrual period than at other times. Birth control pills, which stop the normal cycling of hormones, don't seem to diminish recurrences, but careful studies have not been performed.

Emotional stress may be important for some, but for others stress is unrelated to herpes outbreaks. Trying to force away stress in an attempt to rid oneself of herpes may succeed only in making a lot of new stress. Stress has not been proven to cause herpes to recur. In fact, a recent study was unable to show that stress could be correlated with the timing of a new recurrence. Since herpes itself is stressful, how can we be sure which is the chicken and which is the egg? Herpes is a virus infection, not an episode of the jitters. Reactivation of latent infection in the nervous system is a very complex process that remains poorly understood. Easy answers to tough questions—such as how to control triggers—may be misleading and create false hopes. That is not to say that getting rid of stress is not a good idea. About 75 percent of people who have herpes relate their outbreaks to stress and believe that stress control can lead to herpes control. I encourage everyone to take steps to reduce life's stresses. On the other hand, I encourage everyone to avoid feeling that they have failed or are guilty if efforts at stress control do not reduce herpes outbreaks.

Some people say that sexual intercourse leads to sores. This is also a tough one. Often these are healed sores, usually in the residual redness phase, that have a very thin layer of skin over them that tears easily during intercourse. This occurs mainly in people who have very frequent recurrences. They resume sex after healing, only to find a new sore in the morning. This is frustrating indeed, but sex is probably not the trigger. Rather, sex is the innocent victim of unfortunate circumstance. If you feel that sex triggers recurrences, try waiting a few extra days after healing before resuming sexual contact. It may be the abrasion itself. Try slow and gentle sex and lubricants. Make sure that this really is herpes, by returning to your physician with a new sore. Depending on your individual situation, one of the oral antiviral medicines may be useful (see chapter 11).

Surgery and injury are unavoidable. Sunlight, however, can (and should) be avoided by covering affected areas with clothing or sun-blocking agents. Dr. S. Spruance of the University of Utah recently presented intriguing data on the use of oral acyclovir in patients who were prone to developing sunlight-triggered cold sores. He treated them effectively, before they developed symptoms at all, by predicting that their cold sores would develop after skiing. He went to the ski slopes to get his volunteers. Oral acyclovir is extremely effective at prevention (see chapter 11), much more effective than when it is used after the beginning of even the earliest symptoms of infection. Dr. Stephen Straus took this in a slightly different direction and showed that sun blockers are effective at reducing the incidence of cold sores triggered by the sun. If we could figure out all the triggers in advance of recurrence onset, sun blockers or antiviral agents could be used intermittently to prevent disease. Thus far, however, the only trigger with this predictability level is sunlight on the lip. Since genital herpes is generally covered by clothing, sunlight is not of practical significance in most people. On the other hand, if you like to tan the areas where you get herpes sores, whether type 1 or type 2, you may find that sunlight is a trigger factor for you. You may wish to stop tanning or use suppressive antiviral medication during the summer. You may also wish to consider the fact that ultraviolet light from the sun is dangerous on its own and is a well-known cause of skin cancer and premature aging.

Before you take any medications, including megavitamins, make sure you need them. Never use cortisone creams or any of the derivatives of cortisone (ask your doctor or pharmacist) to treat herpes. If they must be used for another reason, make sure the reason is a good one. Nothing will help a herpes virus live a long, healthy, active life like cortisone. In fact, any ointment other than specific antiviral medication may prolong the duration of sores. People who have readily identifiable triggers may find themselves in situations where triggers are unavoidable. It is rational to consider prophylaxis with antiviral medication for these periods if you wish. You will find more information about this approach in chapter 11.

If I've had a first episode of herpes, will I have a recurrence?

There is no way to predict who will have a recurrence and who will not. Most people will have at least a few. If you have genital herpes simplex virus type 2, you will be more likely to have recurrences than if you have type 1. In fact, type 2 may recur as much as ten to fifteen times as often as type 1 in the genital areas. The reverse is true for facial herpes, where type 1 is far more frequent and recurs much more often. A report by Dr. Lawrence Corey's group at the University of Washington suggests that 84 percent of women and 100 percent of men who have first episodes of type 2 genital herpes have at least one recurrence. For some people, recurrences get milder and less frequent with time, although you should not keep a calendar with the expectation that each recurrence will be shorter than the last. There may be no reduction in the frequency of episodes. The recurrence pattern and severity vary a lot. In fact, if there is one thing you can be sure of, it is that the recurrence pattern will change from time to time. It is this shifting pattern of recurrences that makes the many false cures for herpes seem to work for some people. Such cures turn out to offer no real benefit after rigorous testing. Overall, the average number of recurrences of type 2 genital herpes is about four per year. However, up to 40 percent of people will experience six or more and up to 20 percent of people will experience ten or more symptomatic recurrences in the first year.

Recurrences of herpes can start even as the primary infection heals. Recurrences may overlap, or one may begin as another is ending. They may occur first on the labia and next on the thigh. Episode sites may rotate from one site to another or stay repeatedly in the same place. No treatment during the initial episode has yet been devised that will affect the pattern of future recurrences. Recent studies in animals, however, have suggested that very early treatment with some antiviral medicines may have a long-term benefit. Clinical studies are underway. The reasons for differences in recurrence patterns are not known.

Is it possible to have herpes without any symptoms?

Several studies have shown that antibody directed against type 2 herpes is detected by the Western blot blood test very commonly in people who do not have a history that even suggests genital herpes. Similarly, herpes frequently can be found (if looked for in a research study) in its latent state inside neurons in the sacral ganglia of autopsy cases in which this diagnosis was never suspected and where the person had never reported any symptoms. Furthermore, most people with herpes have not had any contact that they know of with a person with herpes. Similarly, the unknowingly infected sexual partner of someone with a new case of primary genital herpes will usually deny ever having had symptoms of either genital herpes or oral-labial herpes. Even in a private room with a physician listing symptoms, most people will have great difficulty identifying the symptoms of genital herpes until they have understood how mild these sores can be in their recurrent state. As a comparison, the mild mosquito bite that healed a week ago may barely be remembered (if at all) next to the often severe symptoms the primary patient is experiencing. There is often a mistaken expectation that "If the diagnosis is genital herpes in 'my partner with the primary,' then genital herpes in me must look and/or feel the same way." However, genital herpes commonly causes no symptoms at all. In fact, most cases of genital herpes are never recognized unless they are transmitted to someone else, and sometimes not even then. The expectation that a severe infection in one partner will be matched by an infection of equal severity in the other partner is absolutely wrong. Sexually transmitted diseases are most often transmitted from an asymptomatic partner (or sometimes from a partner who does not notice the symptoms) to someone who then may get very severe symptoms. Dr. Anna Wald at the University of Washington recently reported her study of people who tested positive by the Western blot test for type 2 herpes but in whom symptoms of herpes had never been noticed. She found that these people were just as likely to have virus on their genital skin with no symptoms as were people who were already aware of their diagnosis because of sores and symptoms. Sometimes, of course, both partners stay asymptomatic until partners change and a subsequent partner develops more severe symptoms. At this point, patients and couples often become very confused. They ask partners about symptoms and begin to suspect things. Of course, occasionally a partner is lying. But the story of who infected whom can get pretty complicated in a lot of cases. Before you accuse, remember that many people who point fingers at someone for transmitting herpes point in the wrong direction.

The explanation for this confusion is not clear. However, it is easy to see how a mild herpes blister that looks like a pimple or a tiny pinhole might go unnoticed. Even a really severe infection, if localized to the cervix or other internal genital area, may cause no symptoms whatsoever. An infinite number of scenarios to explain asymptomatic transmission can be imagined. For example, a recurrent sore around the anus may cause recurrent rectal itching. This is a symptom that nearly everyone has at one time or another and could easily be passed off as insignificant. Can anyone honestly deny ever having had an itch in the rectum—even one that recurs from time to time?

Does herpes always hurt?

Herpes usually does not hurt much. Severe symptoms are most prominent during the primary infection. Sores that are open and raw are commonly tender or painful to touch. Push a cotton swab on a sore and it will hurt. Urinate on a sore and it will hurt. Itching may be more common than pain during recurrences. Pain is a funny thing. People sense pain differently. Some people with recurrent herpes never feel anything and only know that the herpes is active by looking at the sores. Others are exquisitely aware of the slightest change in their body's chemistry. Regardless, pain is usually not the major problem in coping with recurrent herpes.

On the other hand, patients with strong primary infections may suffer extreme pain for a short time. It may be too painful to urinate, to sit, or to walk. Hospitalization with intravenous antiviral therapy and painkillers may be required. It can be very frightening to imagine this pain recurring every month for a lifetime. Happily, it does not. If you are reading this during your primary, keep in mind that although herpes may recur, it will never again do what it is doing now. Recurrent herpes is not a recurrence of primary herpes. It is generally much milder. Sores are smaller and less painful and are usually gone after several days.

Can herpes cause other kinds of pain?

Because herpes likes nerves, it may cause irritation there. During reactivation (the prodrome phase) the virus travels down the nerve and may cause pain in other areas where the nerve runs. This pain, called *sacral paresthesia*, is often in the leg or buttocks and usually disappears when the prodrome phase is over. Headache may also be a warning sign. Often during a bad primary infection and rarely with a recurrent infection, the reactivating virus travels up the nerve as well as down, finding its way into the central nervous system to cause *meningitis*—an inflammation of the sac around the brain. This inflammation, if caused by herpes, is not generally harmful. It does not damage the nervous system, although it can be quite distressing, resulting in headache, stiff neck, aversion to bright lights, and fever. It does get better quickly. If meningitis occurs, seek the care of a physician so you can be sure that it is just herpes. (Meningitis may require specific therapy.) An unusual, but not rare, complaint after an active recurrence is *postherpetic neuralgia*, or residual pain in the area involved. The skin may feel painful, prickly, itchy, numb, throbbing, cold, hot, or as if it is drawn too tightly. Postherpetic neuralgia generally fades with time. This syndrome is unfortunately very common following herpes zoster (shingles) infection, especially in people who are over the age of fifty or have severe pain when the rash begins. Note that it *follows* active infection and thus does not represent active viral shedding; it is an inactive phase. Other kinds of discomfort occur in some people after a bout of genital herpes. In such cases, shooting pains or aching in the buttock or down the back of one or both legs persists far beyond what one would expect from a simple reactivation of herpes. Presumably, this pain results from a bit of residual nerve damage near the spinal cord, where herpes established its latent infection. If inflammation occurs there, it may be called *radiculitis*. It is usually best to leave the pain untreated and wait for it to fade. However, the physician should decide with you on the best approach. It is important to tell your physician about the symptoms so that he or she can determine that it is only herpes and nothing more serious. Once that is established, there are various treatment options. Sometimes, patients find that trying to control this discomfort with drugs is worse than the problem itself. The only treatment sure not to have adverse effects is no treatment at all. Antiherpesvirus drugs are not especially effective in this setting, although they may be worth a try. Other drugs used for post-herpetic pain include amitryptyline (Elavil), or other tricyclic antidepressants. Neurologists and pain specialists know how to use these drugs. Whatever you do, though, avoid narcotics for post-herpetic pain, if possible. Narcotic analgesics may be very useful for acute pain of herpes—e.g., during or shortly after primary infection, if absolutely necessary. But post-herpetic pain can last quite a long time in some people, and serious drug addiction may result if narcotics are used. Pain and discomfort are common after herpes zoster (shingles) but, luckily, are relatively rare after herpes simplex infection. Get good medical help with this one if it happens to you.

Can herpes make me sterile?

No, but a number of other sexually transmitted infections—for example, *gonorrhea* and *Chlamydia*—can cause sterility. These infections need to be treated with antibiotics in order to stop them from causing harm. The most common warning signs are (male) urethral or (female) vaginal discharge, painful urination, and a painful lower abdomen. These internal genital infections can cause enough inflammation around the ovaries and tubes in a woman to result in scarring, which makes it difficult for the egg to reach the womb. A culture test and examination for pus cells will generally detect these internal genital infections. Many men and women have no symptoms whatsoever of these infections. The doctor who diagnoses herpes should also test for these infections, especially since they are easy to cure with certain antibiotics. In addition, herpes may be confused with *syphilis* and other diseases, even by the most expert, most widely experienced physician. Only laboratory tests can distinguish the different sexually transmitted infections with 100 percent accuracy. Make sure you undergo these tests at least once, usually during your first episode.

Can herpes make me impotent?

Impotence means that a man is unable to obtain and/or sustain an erection when he feels like doing so. Herpes often has a detrimental effect on feeling like it, especially during the period of anger that commonly occurs after people acquire herpes. Emotions such as anger, depression, and hopelessness about having an "incurable" infection commonly influence sexual urges in men and women with herpes. Usually such changes in urges can be corrected by getting over the fear of talking about herpes with your partner. Changes in sexual urges are normal and common. They should not last for a long time.

Severe primary herpes infections, especially in homosexual men with proctitis (rectal-anal infection), may uncommonly result in physical impotence as a result of nerve inflammation. The inflammation leaves after the acute infection and generally does not recur. There are other more common physical causes for impotence, however, such as diabetes mellitus, certain drugs, and hormonal imbalances. If impotence or loss of sexual desire is sustained, you should seek specific medical attention for the problem.

Are cold sores (fever blisters) also herpes?

Yes, for the most part, fever blisters are caused by herpes simplex. The virus is usually (but not always) type 1. Type 2 herpes of the mouth can also cause cold sores, although type 1 is more efficient than type 2 at causing recurrences on the face. (The converse is true for genital sores: type 2 is more efficient than type 1 at causing recurrences on the genitals.) Sores generally look like genital herpes, but they occur on the lip or the skin near the lip. Mouth herpes—like genital herpes—is most often an external disease. The classic cold sore occurs at the vermilion border of the lip— the point where the thin mucous membrane of the mouth changes abruptly into the skin of the face (see figure 12, page 202). Ulcers in the side of the mouth may be herpes but are usually *aphthous ulcers*, which are not infectious. Cracks in the corners of the mouth are usually not caused by herpes.

True cold sores go through a sequence of active phases similar to the sequence already described. The ganglion for cold sore latency is the *trigeminal ganglion*, located inside the skull. The trigeminal sensory nerve comes from this site and supplies sensation to all parts of the face. This nerve is divided into three branches: the *ophthalmic* branch, which provides sensation to the forehead and eye; the *maxillary* branch, which provides sensation to the cheek and side of the nose; and the *mandibular* branch, which provides sensation to the mouth and chin. The mouth is the most common site of herpes recurrences. Virus traveling to the mouth must travel down the mandibular branch of the trigeminal nerve. Regardless of where herpes is inoculated, it will occur along very well defined nerve pathways, following nerve fibers much like a train staying on its track. The track is chosen back at the ganglion level.

Sounds like genital herpes is a bit like a cold sore of the genitals? That's correct. A person with mouth herpes can give a sexual partner genital herpes by having oral-to-genital contact while oral infection is active. The nature of herpes sores and the sites affected depend largely on what gets inoculated where. The primary inoculation site determines where the first lesions will form and which ganglion will subsequently be infected (back at the train station). Recurrence sites, however, are determined by the skin site where the specific nerve fiber (or train track) ends. Usually, the sites of primary inoculation and subsequent recurrence are very closely related, because one nerve ganglion tends to supply sensation to a small, defined area. Occasionally, the two sites may seem to be far apart (e.g., genital herpes recurring on the buttocks), simply because of the nature of nerve branching. The herpes virus does not travel between ganglia, however, so a person with cold sores need not worry that sores will suddenly appear on his or her genitals. If a person gets sores in two sites supplied by two different ganglia, he or she must have been inoculated at both sites. If your cold sores contact the skin of another person during an active phase, the person will become infected and subsequently establish latent infection at the site where the virus was inoculated.

Can I have received my infection months or even years before my first symptoms?

Yes. Although primary genital herpes is usually quite uncomfortable, it often occurs without any symptoms. Unusual symptoms not readily recognized as herpes are also possible. Remember that herpes infections form a spectrum from no symptoms to severe symptoms. Initial infection may pass unnoticed, and recurrent herpes with symptoms may begin later.

A true primary infection, however, with pain, numerous lesions, fever, etc., is unlikely to have been caused by an infection a long time before. The incubation period for primary herpes is between two and thirty days in general. If your first outbreak is mild, it could actually be a recurrent infection—the first recurrence after an asymptomatic primary infection that took place weeks, months, or even years before. In this case, the incubation period is more difficult to pinpoint. If a Western blot test (see chapter 4) is performed early in the first episode, it can identify the episode as either a true primary, a nonprimary initial episode (previous type 1 herpes exposure), or recurrent herpes (previous type 2 herpes exposure). In one study, seventeen of twenty-four people experiencing first episodes of genital herpes were found to have pre-existing antibodies to herpes simplex type 2 and thus were not having true primaries. Most people with pre-existing immunity to herpes at the time of the first clinical episode are experiencing a recurrence after a primary infection that passed unnoticed at some time in the past. Some may be experiencing their first symptoms of a process that began with transmission at a much earlier date. Remember that an incubation period is identifiable only if it is clear that a true primary infection is taking place or if the Western blot blood test proves this fact. By definition, a person with a true primary is seronegative (blood test for herpes completely negative) at the onset of symptoms because that person has not yet had time to raise antibodies against the virus. Separation of a true primary from a nonprimary first episode or recurrence can be very difficult without this blood test.

I often have prodromal symptoms but no sores. What does that mean?

Warning signs without sores probably means reactivation. Most people who have warning symptoms with sores will also have them without sores. The virus has reactivated and may have traveled to the skin, but the body has somehow stopped the infection before it could cause sores. This is very common. In Vancouver, we showed several years ago that about 20 percent of all prodromes will abort without further lesion development, even in the absence of any treatment.

During the prodrome, however, herpes should be considered to be active for a short time. Examine yourself after the warning is over. Sometimes people who believe they do not get sores after the prodrome are not looking closely enough. People with herpes may want to use a mirror, preferably with a well-magnified side, for self-examination. Use a flashlight or another light source that can be brought near to the skin. Remember that sores may vary, may be very small, and may not hurt much. If no signs of herpes occur on the skin, wait a couple of days and resume normal skin contact. If sores develop, follow the phases and wait until the herpes is inactive. It may turn out that many of these *false prodromes* are just that—false. They may be only fleeting neuralgia from the last episode.

False prodromes also occur in some people taking regular oral antiviral medication for prevention of recurrences. Perhaps the recurrent episode begins in the nerve and cycles on but is then aborted before the development of a visible lesion. The significance of these short episodes is unknown. For now, treat them as if they were short recurrences, whether they occur on treatment or off.

Can herpes cause headaches?

Yes, indeed, there is a herpes headache. Headache is very common during a true genital herpes primary infection. Primary herpes is commonly complicated by meningitis, and meningitis headaches are generally quite severe. This is rarely the case in recurrent herpes. Headache may also be associated with other symptoms, such as stiff neck, nausea, and pain from bright light and loud noises. If it occurs during primary herpes, your doctor may choose to perform a lumbar puncture (needle in the low back) so that a sample of spinal fluid can be examined. This is a very safe procedure and generally causes about the same amount of discomfort as a blood test. Some people get a headache from the lumbar puncture test. The test is necessary only where meningitis is considered significant. It is important in some cases to make sure that other causes of meningitis are not present. Herpes meningitis is generally benign; that is, it gets better on its own without treatment and generally does not recur. However, herpes meningitis is often treated with antiviral medications. This is a decision for you and the doctor to make when the diagnosis is considered.

Alternatively, headache may be the symptom of a prodrome. Generally, this headache is mild and has no known cause. In fact, most headaches have no known cause. Being sick with anything can cause a headache. Fever can bring on a headache. Tension from herpes or anything else can bring on a headache. If headaches are very severe, whether you feel they are related to herpes or not, you should discuss the problem with your doctor. Herpes does not generally cause chronic headache.

What other symptoms can herpes cause?

Genital herpes is still a poorly understood disease in many ways. We do not know how many people have it or how many know they have it. We do not know everything it can do. We probably know only some of the symptoms.

The symptoms of herpes are usually related to the sores. If the sores are near the urethra, it may hurt to urinate. If they are on the buttocks, it may hurt to sit. Sometimes, however, herpes causes invisible problems. Some people have recurring leg pain. The pain usually radiates down the back of one leg. It may occur in the thigh. Occasionally, this pain may occur without any sores, like a false prodrome. If it is *episodic* (comes and goes) and is usually followed by sores on the skin, then it is likely a prodrome and should be considered a sign of active herpes. If it is *chronic* (always there or takes weeks to go away), chances are it is not related to herpes. With chronic pain, other causes must be ruled out by a physician. In some cases, pain from herpes can be persistent, long after the virus itself has stopped activity on the skin. Persistent pain after herpes simplex or herpes zoster infection is called *postherpetic neuralgia.* The discomfort of postherpetic neuralgia is usually very similar to the kinds of discomfort experienced during the primary infection; possible symptoms include deep buttock aching, shooting pains down the leg, and numbness in the feet.

During primary infection, any number of unusual things may occur. Primary herpes affects the whole body. Meningitis, as previously described, is common during primary herpes. Very rarely, severe consequences have resulted from herpes, such as severe paralysis from a complication called *transverse myelitis.* Lasting paralysis of muscles from genital herpes is extremely rare, but short-term mild paralysis is not rare during severe primary infection. We have recently seen a patient whose only symptoms during primary genital herpes were leg and bladder weakness with retention of some urine. Absolutely no genital or nongenital lesions were ever seen on this patient. The paralysis was minor and she recovered promptly. Temporary difficulties with urination and weakness in some muscles sometimes occur during primary infection, whether or not sores are present. In fact, minor urinary abnormalities are probably much more common than has been recognized. Where these complications occur, function almost always reverts back to normal after a few weeks.

Occasionally a patient with herpes gets abdominal (stomach) pains from primary herpes. I have been told about patients who have actually undergone surgery for appendicitis only to find out they have primary genital herpes. Gonorrhea and Chlamydia are much more likely causes of abdominal pain than herpes is and are very common causes of *pelvic inflammatory disease* (PID), which often causes lower abdominal pain and may result in sterility. These infections need to be treated by a trained person who must look for them and take a culture in order to identify them.

A curious disease called *erythema multiforme* causes a skin rash with target lesions that look like rings of redness with central color changes (see plate 11, page 100). In addition, the mucous membranes of the mouth, eyes (conjunctiva), or genitals may ulcerate and become painful and raw. Unlike the ulcers of active herpes phases, these ulcers are not infectious. They are generally thought to be a hyperimmune reaction. The body's immune system not only has responded but has overresponded in its efforts to stop the active virus infection during that episode. A few normal cells are damaged by the immune reaction as well, resulting in a rash and ulcers. One of the many causes of erythema multiforme is herpes simplex. Other typical causes include use of certain medications, such as sulfa-containing antibiotics and nonsteroidal anti-inflammatory drugs (NSAIDs) such as aspirin and ibuprofen. Any one individual with herpes is very unlikely to develop this disease, as is any one individual who takes NSAIDs or sulfa drugs. Treatment is sometimes simple and sometimes difficult. Cortisone may be called for and is usually taken by mouth rather than as a cream. The disease may relapse. It needs medical attention. Treatment with antiviral medication is often advisable, and suppression may be indicated in some patients. Discuss treatment with your physician.

Now that I have herpes, am I especially prone to other infections?

Not long ago, doctors were taught that secondary infection of the skin—for example, staph infection or *impetigo*—was a common complication of herpes. This is now known to be false. More than 99 percent of people with herpes have no other infection. Rarely, staph or strep (two common and easily treated bacteria) invade the skin at the site broken by a herpes sore. Where secondary infection occurs, it results in a clinically distinct syndrome different from the usual course of herpes. Patients with these rare complications may develop a syndrome called *cellulitis* (a very uncommon secondary bacterial infection resulting from herpes). A picture of a patient with cellulitis of the groin is shown in plate 12, page 101. The cellulitis rash is quite different from the usual herpes sores. It has a deep red appearance and is often associated with tenderness and fever. Patients with such problems need urgent medical attention and are usually treated with antibiotics in order to clear the secondary bacterial infection. Another type of secondary infection results in each separate vesicle becoming infected and filled with pus (a sticky and thick substance containing inflammatory cells) and often causes an otherwise typical outbreak to persist longer and be more red than usual. Again, antibiotics are indicated.

Because you have acquired one sexually transmitted disease, there is a small statistical risk that you have acquired another at the same time. This possibility does not have to do with your susceptibility but only with your statistical chances of having caught something else. The other common sexually transmitted infections (gonorrhea, Chlamydia, Trichomonas) and those easily confused with herpes because of the way they look (syphilis, chancroid, shingles) should be ruled out. This is discussed in detail in chapter 4.

People whose immunity is compromised by something unrelated to herpes—for example, cancer, lymphoma, leukemia, transplantation, or acquired immune deficiency syndrome (AIDS)—may get herpes simplex infections that do not heal readily, because their immunity problems make them more susceptible to problematic herpes.

Recent studies have shown that there is one correlation between herpes and human immunodeficiency virus (HIV). Specifically, people with herpes (as well as virtually any other genital ulcer disease) are statistically more likely to have acquired human immunodeficiency virus infection than are people who do not have any genital ulcer disease. There are two possible explanations. First, both infections are sexually transmitted, so it is not surprising that they may be found together. Second, the immune cells that fight off infection with any genital ulcer disease are highly concentrated at the site of a sore or genital ulcer. In the base of the ulcer, fighter cells called "helper" lymphocytes or CD4+ cells work to protect the body from further invasion by whichever infection is causing the genital ulcer. Such cells are the main target cells for attack by the human immunodeficiency virus. So, if HIV is present during sexual contact and if the cells containing this virus find a genital ulcer conveniently available, then HIV can find ready entry into its prime target cell. In fact, virtually all diseases that lead to genital ulcers result in the same situation—an easy target. Thus, even though there is some association of these two viruses, one does not cause the other. To get HIV, you have to be exposed to HIV. If, when you are exposed to HIV, you have an unhealed genital ulcer, your risk of actually acquiring HIV on that occasion goes up somewhat. But having herpes alone does not cause HIV infection. In fact, people who are careful about avoiding herpes transmission do not have sexual contact during the active ulcer stage anyway.

Herpes infection might actually lessen the risk of HIV infection in many people; people who acquire herpes tend to reduce their exposure risk to HIV by reducing their numbers of sexual partners and adopting safer sexual practices. Dr. Suzanne Kroon of Denmark has called this change in lifestyle, "increasing the quality control [of partners]." It is one of the real benefits of having genital herpes, and it could conceivably save your life. People with herpes who elect to ignore these risk factors do run the risk of acquiring HIV and, if exposed, are approximately twice as susceptible to actually becoming infected compared with people who do not have recurrent genital sores.

4
Genital Herpes:
The Diagnosis

Choice is future oriented and never fully expressed in present action. It requires what is most distinctive about human reasoning: intention—the capacity to envisage and to compare future possibilities, to make estimates, sometimes to take indirect routes to a goal or to wait.

—SISSELA BOK
Secrets: On the Ethics of Concealment and Revelation

How is the diagnosis made?

In some situations, genital herpes may be a simple diagnosis for the general practitioner. In others, it may elude the specialist. When symptoms and signs of herpes are "classical"—that is, when exposure is known to have taken place and painful clustered vesicles (blisters) or ulcers have developed on a red, inflamed base—the clinical diagnosis is clear-cut. Recurrences make herpes even more likely. Then, the virus itself is detected by a culture test from one of the sores, confirming the diagnosis. In order to make sure that no other diseases accompany herpes, tests for syphilis, gonorrhea, Chlamydia, Trichomonas, HIV, and yeast are also performed.

On the other hand, some people with genital herpes have mild intermittent symptoms. The only sore may be a single pinpoint ulcer on the labia that lasts for a few days, occurs every six months, and does not hurt at all. The diagnosis may not even occur to the patient or the physician. A virus culture test to detect herpes in the sore should be performed during an active phase of infection. If the test is positive, herpes is likely to be the cause of the sore. A positive culture for herpes simplex virus from the skin means that you have herpes. The virus culture is so reliable, it is called the gold standard for this infection.

If the test is negative, however, herpes may or may not be the cause of the problem. Consider the phases of herpes (discussed in chapter 3). Was the test obtained during an active period? If not, it can be expected to be negative, even if herpes is the problem. Even if the period was an active one, quite often herpes virus is not recoverable. How was the test obtained? Was the doctor's office far away from the laboratory? If so, the virus may not have survived the trip. How experienced is the laboratory? This varies. Some laboratories save money by dividing up clinical samples into extremely small samples, so that they can actually perform 96 different viral culture tests on the surface of one plastic plate. Such cost-savers will reduce the sensitivity of the test. Most quality laboratories are certified by the College of American Pathologists (CAP) or whatever governing body for accreditation is applicable in your area. Even under ideal circumstances, virus recovery in the laboratory after only one try is not always possible.

If you suspect herpes and your doctor agrees, your best bet is to return again for virus culture at the first sign of recurrence. The earlier the specimen is obtained, the better the chance of an accurate test. In my experience, two visits will suffice, if the visits are early. If herpes is suspected and cultures are negative, it is probably best to try to obtain a Western blot (blood) test. This test is described later in this chapter.

I have been exposed to someone who has herpes. Should I go to my doctor now for a test?

This is an increasingly common question. It is also a difficult problem. If you have been exposed to someone with herpes, the person's herpes may have been active or inactive.

If your partner's herpes was in an inactive stage, your risk is very low. If no symptoms develop, you do not need to do anything. Nothing will almost certainly be what continues to happen unless you become exposed, in the future, to an active infection.

If your partner's infection was in an active stage, you may have come into contact with the virus. Whether or not you will develop herpes depends on several factors.

Was there virus present? The active stages are a good guess for when exposure risk is high, but often sores contain no living virus. If sores were active, you may have been infected, but not necessarily so.

The number of virus particles (inoculum) is important. If the inoculum that made contact was very high, then infection is more likely. If virus was present in very small amounts, infection is less likely.

Where did inoculation take place? Was this contact through thin skin—for instance, on the genitals? Were there cuts on the skin? Was contact prolonged? Did a long time elapse before washing the area? Are you female? (Women have about three to four times more risk of being infected than men.) All of these things might increase the chance for any virus to transfer from one person to another.

Several other "host factors" also play a role. If you already have antibody to type 1 herpes simplex virus (more than half of North Americans have this without knowing it), a higher dose of herpes simplex virus type 2 is probably required to result in infection. If you already have herpes simplex virus type 2 (about 20 percent of North American people have this antibody without knowing it), you may not really even be at any substantial risk of catching genital herpes at all, since you already have it. The immune system may also be an important factor in some ways we do not understand.

Whether or not you develop symptoms of herpes will determine the type of diagnostic test you require. If no symptoms are present, only the Western blot test can be used to diagnose genital herpes. This is one occasion when you need to be very careful about what information the doctor has when the diagnosis is made or excluded. It might be a good idea to show your doctor this chapter to make sure that you are both talking about the same issues. By performing a history and physical examination and cultures for virus, the doctor can rule out problems other than genital herpes. If you have symptoms, this examination may tell you what you do have. Examination and culture alone, however, cannot exclude what you do not have. In other words, if you do not have an active sore at the time you are examined, the doctor cannot correctly conclude, on this basis, that you do not have genital herpes. The same is true of a partner. If a viral culture test for herpes comes up positive, of course, that does correctly diagnose herpes. A negative culture test, though, does not exclude the diagnosis. Why? Because herpes is recurrent, with a lot of inactive and unpredictable episodic time between relapses. The examination and viral culture test would come up negative most of the time even in a person who has herpes, because the virus is inactive most of the time. If symptoms develop—e.g. vaginal discharge, sores, unexplained tenderness of the genitals, redness, pimples, or swollen lymph nodes—then go to the doctor without delay. If there is no other obvious cause for the symptoms, and exposure to herpes is likely, inform the doctor and ask for a herpes culture. Go early, when symptoms are present. Waiting it out does not help. Herpes will go away on its own, only to probably return again. If you want to know (and it is your responsibility to know), go to the doctor when symptoms first appear.

The most advanced blood test for herpes, currently available in a few centers, is the *Western blot test*. If a visible sore is present, this test is unnecessary, since the virus culture test not only is the gold standard but is also cheaper and is often a better, more direct means of detecting the presence of virus. The blood test is described later in this chapter. The blood test to rule out herpes after a possible exposure may be especially useful, since sores often do not develop and people still want to know if they were exposed. The blood test cannot tell you where you were exposed, but it can be used to determine if type 2 herpes simplex virus infection is present. The type-specific antibody test must be performed at least twelve weeks after a possible exposure in order to be reasonably sure that a negative result truly means that you probably have not acquired herpes. In the best hands, this test is very accurate, but no test is 100 percent sensitive. Occasionally, even the best test misses the mark. In some people, it takes several weeks to convert to a positive. The type-specific test is just coming into its own, however. The test is difficult to get. It is the best test for this situation, currently, but different labs do things differently. Before having the test done at a laboratory, be sure that the test:

1. is type-specific by testing at least for *glycoprotein G-2* (gG-2) by Western blot or some other proven method and,

2. is well controlled. What is the lab's sensitivity rate? (In other

words, how often does this lab come up with a negative test that is falsely negative (incorrect)?) The best Western blot tests are close to 99 percent accurate. Ask your health care provider about this.

You might consider taking a course of one of the oral antiviral agents against herpes because of virus exposure before developing symptoms (see chapter 11) if: 1.) you feel your exposure to an active herpes sore was fairly certain, 2.) you feel that you may be susceptible to getting herpes (do not already have the same type of herpes as your partner), and 3.) your exposure happened within the past few days (preferably fewer than three days).

How is the diagnosis proven?

The best way to prove that herpes is present, regardless of how sure it looks, is with a test that shows herpes simplex virus to be present in a sore. The most sensitive test (the most likely to show positive when it is herpes) is a culture test. Since virus lives inside cells, a few of the cells from a sore must be taken and sent for culture. A wet cotton or Dacron swab is rolled into a sore, put into a special salt solution, and sent to the laboratory.

At the lab, some of the fluid is removed and placed onto healthy human cells that are kept growing in tubes. The cells are called a tissue culture. Once virus is placed onto the tissue culture, it is called a virus culture. The laboratory technician keeps the cells growing at body temperature in an incubator and, during the next several days, removes the culture from the incubator and places it under the microscope. If the cells remain healthy, the culture is negative. If the cells become sick from herpes, they will round up and group themselves together. This change in appearance is called the *cytopathic effect* (CPE). An area of herpes infection of cells called *fibroblasts* is shown in figure 8. Note the long, pointed, wispy appearance of the normal cells, on the upper left, compared to the sick-looking swollen cells where the virus is growing, to the left of the bracket.

Once the CPE has occurred, the technician puts a small number of cells from the tube onto a slide and adds a herpes simplex antibody to the slide. The antibody is usually attached to a chemical that fluoresces (emits light) under ultraviolet (UV) light. If the cells fluoresce, the changes in the cells must have been caused by herpes simplex. A positive fluorescence test is shown in plate 4, page 97. The bright areas on the cells are fluorescing because herpes antibody is stuck to the virus on the cell. Note the apple green rim containing the fluorescent dye linked to the antibody.

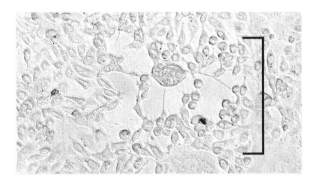

Figure 8: Microscopic appearance of cells affected by herpes simplex virus. Normal cells in culture are altered by the infection taking place in the test tube. Cells are swollen and fused. This is called the cytopathic effect (or CPE) and is suggestive of herpes simplex infection.

Several other methods of diagnosis may also be used. If fluid is present—e.g., inside a vesicle—the virus may be seen under an electron microscope, a very powerful (and very expensive) piece of equipment about the size of a small car. An experienced and capable technician must operate the machine. Identification of herpes-like particles is truly an art (see figure 3, page 32). Interpretation may be very difficult and, unfortunately, occasionally misleading. All herpes viruses look the same under the electron microscope. Nobody can say, just from this test, if the virus is type 1 or type 2 or even if it is shingles. Furthermore, even though the machine is powerful, it is not sensitive. One must have a lot of virus in a very carefully collected specimen in order to obtain a positive electron microscope test. One must further have great faith in the talents of the technician.

The fluorescent antibody technique described above for cells in culture can also be performed directly on clinical specimens, or a smear from the sore can be put onto a microscope slide and examined directly (a Pap smear). If herpes causes giant cells to form, the giant cells can be seen in the microscope directly. Special stains can be done on the slide, which is then called a *Tzanck smear.*

The smears, the fluorescence, and the electron microscopy tests are quick tests. Others are being developed, as well. In general, compared to culture tests these quick answer tests sacrifice accuracy for speed or convenience. A herpes diagnostic kit called Herpchek, made by Dupont, is very easy for labs to use and is just as sensitive as the culture test. This test is very accurate, but it does not "type" the virus (i.e. determine if it is herpes simplex virus type 1 or type 2). It is called an *enzyme immunoassay* (EIA). EIA is a method of testing either blood or a swab for herpes. The method may be adequate for a swab test but not yet for a type-specific blood test.

Many laboratories now use an extremely sensitive test called the *polymerase chain reaction test* (PCR). PCR is far more sensitive than a culture test and can detect even a few molecules of herpes DNA on the skin. It is currently three to four times as expensive as a culture test and about twice the expense of a Western blot.

Which test to do depends on the situation. Sometimes it is necessary to do more than one type of test. Each of these methods provides direct evidence of herpes infection and, if positive, proves that herpes is present. A negative result on one specific virus test does not prove that herpes is not present. If there is a negative finding, the Western blot test described below is the best way to go.

Is there a blood test for herpes?

Can I take a blood test to accurately determine the presence of herpes? Yes. In fact, this test has markedly improved physicians' ability to properly counsel both patients and their partners. Herpes blood tests measure the body's immune response against the virus. Without infection, there is no specific reaction to the virus. In contrast, shortly after a true viral infection, the body responds to fight the infection. The herpes blood test measures that response by measuring the body's antibody to herpes. All herpes antibody tests do essentially the same thing. They do not directly measure virus. They measure, instead, the body's reaction to the virus. To look directly for virus, one must test a sore containing virus and grow the virus in the laboratory. This has the advantage of determining not only the virus and its type but also what the sores look like and whether or not they contain virus. Because of its dependence on the active sore, however, the virus culture test also has some key disadvantages. To get a positive test from a culture, a person with herpes must have symptoms. Without symptoms, there is nothing to test. Furthermore, the sore must be tested at just the right moment. If it is too early, there may not be an adequate quantity of infected cells. If it is too late in the course of a recurrence, the virus may have already been killed by the body's defenses.

An accurate blood test for herpes antibody has been needed for a long time. An accurate blood test, such as the Western blot, could be used to help diagnose herpes in people who do not even get sores and in people who get them only rarely. People who might want such a test would include the partner who is asymptomatic but may have been the source of herpes. Other blood test candidates would be the person with only one past episode whose culture was lost on the way to the lab, people who think they have been exposed to herpes but are not sure, and couples who want to give up safer sex precautions. If you have no trouble getting a viral test directly from a sore during an active phase, then that is the preferred approach. But if this presents difficulty for any reason, the Western blot is preferred.

Most commercial herpes antibody (blood) tests are not type-specific. All they can tell you is that you have *herpes* of some sort. (Positive results on these tests are common since 50 to 80 percent of people over twenty have antibodies to the herpes simplex virus.) Unfortunately, many of the commercial blood tests advertised as *type-specific* widely available to doctors are not very accurate at doing what they claim to do—determining whether you have type 1 or type 2 herpes. Even though they may be based on type-specific laboratory markers, most of them correlate only poorly to the actual clinical situation. These tests (which include enzyme immunoassays [EIA], complement fixation tests, and tests for immunoglobulin M [IgM]) are simply not yet sufficiently accurate for a proper diagnosis of genital herpes. This will probably change in the future. These tests *are* still clinically useful at present, however, in that they can be used to detect antibodies to herpes in the blood and, therefore, determine whether a first episode of genital herpes—already diagnosed by viral culture and typing—is a true primary or a nonprimary.

Accurate type-specific antibody tests that have recently been developed test directly for the body's reaction (antibody production) against a type-2-specific glycoprotein, G-2 (gG-2). Very few laboratories test directly for this antibody, since commercial test kits are not routinely available for this purpose. Until new tests replace the old tests, you and your physician will have to interpret information obtained very carefully. This section is an attempt to guide you through the jungle.

The *Western blot* (also called immunoblot) test has been used for diagnosis of viral infections since 1979. This test was first adapted for use with herpes simplex virus by Dr. David Bernstein in 1985. Most of the work perfecting the use of this test for clinical diagnosis has been conducted by Dr. Rhoda Ashley and her colleagues at the University of Washington. They first reported their method in 1988. Using their test, it is possible to determine from a blood sample whether a person has ever been infected with herpes simplex virus type 1, with herpes simplex virus type 2, with both, or with neither. The Western blot is by far the best understood and most reliable type-specific antibody test.

To perform a Western blot, proteins made by herpes simplex virus are separated and sorted using a technique known as electrophoresis. The viral proteins are first put on a polyacrylamide gel which resembles overly-dried Jello. By running a current through the gel, the proteins are separated into a pattern of bands unique to the viral type (herpes type 1 and type 2 have their own distinctive pattern, see figure 9).

The proteins are then transferred onto a strip of nitrocellulose paper that binds them tightly, preserving the distribution pattern. Blood samples are then tested using strips specific for both herpes simplex virus type 1 and herpes simplex virus type 2. If antibodies to herpes simplex virus are present in the blood, they will bind to the proteins on the strips in the same pattern of bands. The bands are then visualized using radioactive or chemical methods.

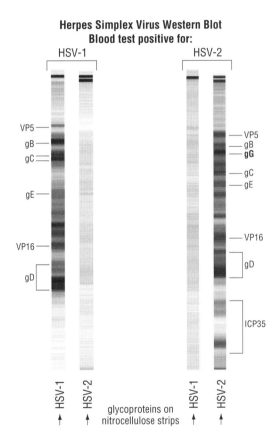

Figure 9: The Western blot test.

The laboratory uses several different controls to be sure that a pattern is clearly specific to type 2 herpes simplex virus. Once all those criteria are met, the test is called positive. For example, if there is a predominance of binding to the type 1 strip or if there are bands of antibody bound to both strips but none are stuck to the gG-2 band (found only in type 2 virus), then there is antibody only against herpes simplex virus type 1. If there is a predominance of binding to the type 2 strip, with specific binding to the gG-2 band, then there is herpes simplex virus type 2 infection. If there is binding to both strips plus the gG-2 band, then there is probably a mixed infection (type 1 and type 2).

Highly skilled interpretation is necessary, and each specimen has to be individualized. Often several readers interpret each blot to ensure accuracy. Mixed infections (type 1 and type 2 together) are sometimes very difficult to interpret. To determine if there is any antibody to herpes simplex virus type 2 present, the laboratory may need to clear the blood sample of all of its antibody to herpes simplex virus type 1. To do this, the laboratory first mixes the sample with a purified protein mixture from type 1 virus. Any type 1 antibodies in the blood will then bind to the proteins. The mixture is then cleared from the blood and the remaining sample is retested against a herpes simplex virus type 2 strip to look for the band binding to gG-2. In this way, the laboratory expert can use a combination of patterns and other characteristics to interpret the response, minimizing the chance of a mistake.

Using these steps, there is virtually no chance of an error that shows a positive antibody to herpes simplex virus type 2 where none exists. On the other hand, there is always a small possibility that an antibody to herpes simplex virus type 2 will go undetected by this method. This could happen in the case of a recently infected person who has not yet had time to produce a lot of antibodies. In some cases, a person may take as long as twelve or sixteen weeks to develop antibodies, especially if the primary infection was treated with an effective medication. Occasionally, a person with culture-proven, long-lasting, recurrent type 2 herpes will still have a negative Western blot—presumably because they just do not make enough of the antibody. It's estimated that this occurs only about 1 percent of the time. This test is very sensitive, but does not detect every situation where genital herpes is present. In the hands of an expert laboratory, it is also very accurate, with virtually no incorrect positives made. If a person is tested more than twelve to sixteen weeks after the suspected exposure and the test is negative, then it is very likely that infection by type 2 herpes virus did not take place. However, no test is absolutely without fault. This test—like all tests—should be discussed by you and your physician in the context of all other clinical information, so that everyone understands the subtle details.

Other tests for gG-2 are also available in some research laboratories. These tests can determine whether there has been infection with herpes simplex virus type 2, but they do not determine whether there has been infection with type 1. EIA tests are technically much easier to perform than the Western blot, with much of the assay actually done by machine. Research tests of this type have been successfully used, with one described from Atlanta, one from California, another from Sweden, and an adaptation from Australia. Unfortunately, commercial EIA kit assays for antibody to gG-2 are not yet available. This situation is very likely to change soon.

For now, be especially careful to check with your physician as to which test is being ordered and how it will be interpreted. If possible, do this before being tested. The situation can be very confusing, because if your physician has ordered a so-called type-specific EIA test that does not check for antibody against gG-2 or some other type 2 viral glycoprotein, then the test may be of no value. So-called type-specific tests that often give misleading test results are most often reported as "type 2:type 1 ratios." You may want to ask your doctor to arrange for the Western blot test instead.

It is probably best to give some examples of real cases where I have found the Western blot test to be especially useful. Test results will be different for each person depending upon their own experience. These specific examples are selected because they are particularly illustrative.

Example 1: A person with a history of genital herpes was seen twelve months after recovering from genital sores diagnosed by visual examination as probable primary genital herpes. A virus culture performed at the time was negative, but the person's physician explained that a negative result does not rule out genital herpes. At that time, the person was advised to return with an active episode for repeat culture, but no recurrences were detected. The patient has had one monogamous relationship, which started just before the so-called primary infection, with a partner who has no history of genital symptoms. They commonly practice oral-genital sex. Neither partner has cold sores.

Serology (blood antibody test) result: Both partners are positive for herpes simplex virus type 1 and negative for herpes simplex virus type 2.

Interpretation: Blood test results must be interpreted in the clinical setting. It is likely that the patient's partner does not have genital herpes. The patient's genital sores may have been a primary genital episode but, if so, probably resulted from oral-genital transmission of herpes simplex virus type 1 from the partner. Regardless, the prognosis for a continuing low genital recurrence rate is excellent. Alternatively, these blood test results could be consistent with both patient and partner having been exposed on the face to cold sores at some time in their lives, while neither has genital herpes at all. (The patient's sores may have been something else.) A third explanation is that the partner transmitted herpes simplex virus type 1 to the patient by genital contact with asymptomatic genital herpes simplex virus type 1 sores. Alternative diagnoses to the patient's primary herpes diagnosis should be considered, especially if symptoms recur frequently. The serology test is only supportive evidence for the diagnosis. It does not determine where on the body exposure has taken place, and it must be interpreted cautiously and in connection with the clinical picture. This patient with genital sores should be quite certain that other causes of genital ulcers have been ruled out, since the precise diagnosis is not yet known. In this case, the serology test has helped to rule out some things but has not specifically confirmed the clinical problem. It is very important that this patient be tested to make sure that syphilis did not cause the ulcer, since syphilitic ulcers, left untreated, will improve and then remain dormant only to cause damage later on. The result above could be consistent with both patient and partner having immunity to herpes simplex virus type 1 from asymptomatic mouth cold sores and with one partner having transmitted syphilis that has never been diagnosed or treated. Without a test, nobody will know.

Alternative serology result: Both partners are negative for both herpes simplex virus type 1 and herpes simplex virus type 2.

Interpretation: The initial diagnosis of genital herpes was probably incorrect. An alternative diagnosis should be considered, but if the infection remains inactive, the cause may never come to light. The syphilis test discussed above is crucial, although the result is likely to be negative. If sores are recurrent, one or more specialist physicians should be involved to try to sort out the proper diagnosis.

Alternative serology result: The partner is positive for both herpes simplex virus type 1 and herpes simplex virus type 2. The patient is positive for herpes simplex virus type 2 only.

Interpretation: The initial diagnosis of genital herpes is correct. The person has had primary genital herpes simplex virus type 2 infection, and the source was probably the current partner, who is asymptomatic. Recurrences may be mild but should be expected.

Example 2: Type 2 genital herpes was proven by viral cultures in a person having a clinical first episode of genital herpes. The non-type-specific antibody test performed at the outset of this episode was positive, showing that this was a nonprimary first episode. The patient had two different sexual partners around the time of the first episode. One of the partners is interested in finding out whether he or she was the source of infection.

Serology result: The partner is positive for both herpes simplex virus type 1 and herpes simplex virus type 2.

Interpretation: The partner has genital herpes and also has been exposed to herpes simplex virus type 1. The serology test does not determine where and when the infection took place. The seropositive partner may indeed have been the source of herpes for this patient, but he or she is not the only possible source partner here. The patient could have had herpes for a while and only now be manifesting symptoms. Delving more deeply into the symptoms may help work this one out. However, most herpes is asymptomatic, so a positive test for herpes simplex virus type 2 antibody is expected more than half the time in persons with more than ten or so lifetime partners. The patient may have been positive for a long time before any contact with this current partner.

Example 3: As in example 2, type 2 genital herpes was proven in a patient with a clinical first episode. However, in this example, the early non-type-specific antibody test was negative, showing that this was a true primary first episode. Again, the patient had two different sexual partners around the time of the first episode. One of the partners is interested in finding out whether he or she was the source of infection.

Serology result: The partner is positive for herpes simplex virus type 1 and herpes simplex virus type 2.

Interpretation: This partner has exactly the same blood test results as the partner in example 2, but, in this case, the patient had a known true primary. That changes the interpretation somewhat. This partner has type 2 genital herpes and is the likely source of the primary in the patient. However, it is still possible that this partner may not have exposed the patient with primary infection. The other partner could be seropositive also and could have been the one whose herpes was active recently. In fact, it is possible that the patient with the primary could have exposed this partner to herpes for the first time, rather than the other way around. If this partner's serology test was actually taken *during* the primary infection, however, this would show that the partner was not exposed primarily to herpes by the patient, since it would take at least one or two weeks (or as long as twelve to sixteen weeks) to become seropositive.

If the story were a bit different, and the patient with the proven primary infection had had only one source partner during the month before symptoms developed, a positive serologic test for the same viral type in the partner would confirm unequivocally that the single partner was the source. However, this serology in the partner may be unnecessary, since having only one partner before developing a proven primary is strong enough evidence that that partner is the source—as long as the first clinical outbreak is actually proven to be a true primary (started out seronegative).

Now that you think you have figured this all out, think of this. It is in fact possible for a partner to be truly seronegative and transmit herpes. How? Remember that it takes a while for blood antibodies to be raised (seroconversion). If the source partner has just been infected for the first time from a different source (i.e., a different sexual partner), then he or she would not yet have converted to seropositive. In fact, people who are in the early stages of a primary infection are in their most infectious stage ever, whether or not they are showing any symptoms of herpes, since early primary infection is the time when viral shedding on mucosal surfaces is the highest.

Example 4: A patient keeps going to the physician because of recurrent genital ulcers, which look like cuts or cracks along the lines of skin folds. Cultures for herpes simplex have been taken repeatedly from sores that often have a creamy discharge. None have been positive. Simultaneous cultures of samples from the base of the sores showed only yeast on a few occasions. The physician thinks this is probably herpes but is not certain.

Serology result: The patient is negative for both herpes simplex virus type 1 and herpes simplex virus type 2.

Interpretation: This patient has no evidence of genital herpes and is probably experiencing genital ulcers because of recurrent yeast infections which require a very different type of treatment. These negative tests usually mean that there is about 99 percent chance that there has been no exposure to either herpes simplex virus type 1 or herpes simplex virus type 2. An alternative explanation is that the person was exposed less than twelve weeks ago and has not yet shown the seroconversion. There is a small (approximately 1 percent) chance that this person actually has genital herpes simplex virus type 2 herpes despite the negative serologic test. The small chance of a false negative test is likely to get even smaller in the next few years as the technology for this test continues to improve.

Example 5: A couple in a long-term relationship wish to be tested for herpes. One partner has genital herpes simplex virus type 2 proven by viral culture. The other partner is asymptomatic, although they have been together for several years. The partner wants to know if he or she is still at risk of getting genital herpes.

Serology result: There is virtually never a need to perform a Western blot in a person with viral culture proven type 2 herpes simplex virus infection, since the viral culture (if it is positive) tells you even more. That is, it identifies the infection and the site of the infection. However, the partner should be tested. In this case, she or he is seropositive for herpes simplex virus type 2.

Interpretation: This partner has genital herpes. He or she may have had genital herpes at the time the couple met, or asymptomatic transmission may have taken place at some point in their relationship. Either way, there is very little risk of the partner catching a second infection with type 2 herpes virus. This couple can relax some of their concerns about transmission of genital herpes since both already have proven infections. While there are cases of second viral strain transmission, the chance that that will occur appears to be low, although definitive studies have not been performed.

Summary

Type-specific serology testing is changing the way genital herpes is diagnosed in some cases. It is especially useful in unusual presentations of herpes and in asymptomatic cases. People with genital sores will still want to have a viral culture test from a sore for confirmation and typing. The culture test is more direct and less expensive and provides information about the sore and the symptoms. The blood test may (and often does) come up positive in people with absolutely no symptoms of genital herpes. If you have a clear positive viral culture test that is typed (type 1 versus type 2) there is almost never a reason to bother getting a Western blot also.

A negative Western blot test means that genital herpes is very unlikely, although there is still a small chance of a false negative. A positive test for type 2 herpes strongly suggests the diagnosis of genital herpes, although the test does not determine the site of infection. People with type 2 herpes infection in any site on the body will have a positive test, although most type 2 herpes is sexually transmitted and usually affects areas on or near the genitals or anus. There are obvious exceptions, however. Furthermore, since genital herpes can be caused by type 1 herpes simplex virus, a negative test for type 2 does not rule out genital herpes: it only makes type 2 genital herpes very unlikely, as long as the twelve to sixteen weeks waiting period has passed. It may take up to twelve to sixteen weeks after infection for the serology test to show positive. Any test result should be interpreted with your physician.

What type of doctor should I go to?

You may wish to start with your family doctor or internist. Find out whether your symptoms suggest herpes. If you need more detailed answers to your questions, ask to be referred to a clinic for sexually transmitted diseases or to a specialist in the area. Your physician should be able to guide you to a gynecologist, a dermatologist, a urologist, a specialist in infectious diseases, or someone who has some special experience with herpes. It matters little how much or what type of special training the physician or health practitioner has. In some areas, it is very common for people with genital problems to go directly to a specialist; in other areas, it is common to go to a clinic, where most care is provided by a nurse or a physician's assistant. In most cases, a superspecialist is not required to get proper diagnosis, treatment, and counseling for sexually transmitted diseases. It is information and accuracy that you need. Only a trained professional can arrange for the other tests you will need to be sure you have nothing else that requires specific treatment.

Expect to be fully questioned, often about private matters. Your physician needs to know answers to (and usually needs to ask you directly) very personal questions you may never have been asked before. To provide you with some idea about the types of questions the practitioner should be asking, a questionnaire from the Viridae Herpes Clinic is included as an appendix in the back of this book. The questionnaire is for you to use if you wish when you go to your doctor. Feel free to make a copy; fill it out carefully and give it to your physician or health care provider. I am not suggesting that every health care provider should be using this same approach. The form in the appendix is for women who are pregnant. We use slightly different forms for non-pregnant women and for men. There would be additional (or different) questions we would ask in these situations, of course. However, your health care provider should be asking you at least in general terms about some of the areas covered in the questionnaire. In my opinion, the most important areas include the following:

1. Your history of herpes, including the first episode—duration, appearance, symptoms associated with it, treatment of it, tests done to determine the cause.

2. Your sexual history—i.e., number of sexual partners, sexual preference, other sexually transmitted disease risk factors, risk factors for acquiring AIDS.

3. Your coping mechanisms—e.g., excessive moodiness or black moods, feeling of being depressed, thoughts about suicide, waking up during the night, thinking a lot about death.

4. Your history of other medical conditions and treatments.

5. How herpes is affecting your life in general and specifically your relationship(s).

After your physician has taken a full history about you and your herpes, you should be fully examined. A woman should have a full external and internal genital examination, at least once after the onset of her herpes (and also as a regular part of her yearly routine physical, of course). Men should be examined externally and should also, in most cases, have a urethral swab or urine test for other STDs. Examination of the area around the rectum is also important for both men and women. A full examination may not seem very dignified, but if your health care provider fails to make the right diagnosis about your infection because an examination was replaced by counseling, then you have been done no favor.

In addition to a complete history and physical examination and laboratory tests, your physician should offer specific advice about herpes. Herpes is very common, but, even today, many people with herpes find going to their doctor unsatisfactory. In a recent study from the American Social Health Association in the United States, people with herpes stated that their first health care provider had failed to take a proper sexual history or ask about personal issues in more than half of all cases!

As a health care consumer, you may need to shop around a bit, but you should get your history taken, your physical examination performed, your questions answered. Your health care provider should be comfortable with you (and you with him or her), with the diagnosis of herpes, and with your partner if you wish your partner to be present. The health care provider should arrange for follow-up if this is your primary, in order to be certain all the information and medicine did their work.

Does it matter if the herpes is type 1 or type 2?

As a general rule, herpes simplex is herpes simplex. Usually, type 1 causes oral, lip, and facial herpes, while type 2 causes genital herpes. However, type 1 may cause genital herpes and type 2 may cause oral herpes. In general, however, in North America, over 90 percent of *recurrent* genital herpes is caused by type 2. This continues to be true because type 2 herpes simplex virus infection recurs much more efficiently on the genital area compared with type 1. In part, this is probably due to the efficiency of type 2 herpes in attaching itself to nerve cells (neurons) in the sacral ganglia. In animal models, nerve cells from these areas are much easier targets for type 2 than for type 1. More sacral ganglionic neurons become latently infected and more are likely to reactivate with type 2 than with type 1.

By contrast, *primary* genital infection from a type 1 infection is very common. Primary infection results from external inoculation of skin cells from the infected skin of another. Latent infection takes place as a result. The opposite situation takes place with recurrent infection, where sores result from *reactivation* of latent neuron infection in the same person. In fact, nearly half of true primary genital herpes is now caused by type 1. Type 1 genital primaries are on the rise for a number of reasons. First of all, primary infection depends on how much virus is present in the skin of the source partner during contact. Type 1 contact potential may be increasing in adulthood because oral sex is becoming more common and is rarely a protected sexual practice (using latex barriers, for example). The vast majority of type 1 genital herpes results from unprotected oral-genital sex. Even more importantly, the level of our immunity to type 1 oral-labial herpes in adults is now much lower than it ever was. This is, of course, all the fault of our parents! They were much more aware of and careful with their cold sores than previous generations were. Their careful hygiene markedly reduced the incidence of facial type 1 herpes in children. However, these precautions have also had the side effect of leaving us significantly more susceptible to both type 1 and type 2 herpes simplex virus transmission as adults.

Therapy is now available for treatment of herpes infections. Some of the therapy being developed may be type-specific. If type-specific therapy becomes a clinical reality (which is some time off), then typing before treatment will become absolutely necessary. Some laboratories now do herpes typing routinely. In the recent past, typing was a difficult thing to do well, but the laboratory methods for proper typing are now much easier, and they will become easier yet in the very near future.

Even before the era of type-specific therapy, however, the virus should be typed accurately during the very first episode of genital herpes. Type 1 and type 2 have very different outcomes regarding recurrence frequency and very different habits regarding methods of transmission. These differences can be quite important. For example, if a first genital outbreak occurs in a young child, the possibility of sexual abuse should be investigated by the authorities. If the child has type 1 genital herpes, it becomes possible or perhaps likely, that he or she acquired herpes through nonsexual contact. But while it is possible to conceive of a nonsexual mode of transmission for type 2 genital herpes to a child, those situations must be rare. It is also important to know your herpes type because most primary outbreaks caused by type 1 will not lead to frequent recurrences. Type 1 recurrent herpes generally occurs far less often than type 2. Thus, it is reassuring to find out during the primary episode which type you have, should it turn out to be type 1. Another reason to find out which type you have is that if it is type 1, it was probably transmitted through oral-genital contact; if so, it is likely (but not certain) that your sexual partner got herpes in a nonsexual way, because most type 1 herpes is transmitted through mouth/facial contact in childhood. Type 1 genital herpes is also less frequently shed without symptoms compared with type 2. If transferred during childbirth to cause neonatal herpes, type 1 can cause serious infections for the neonate, but is less likely to lead to long-term problems in the infant following recovery. On the other hand, since recurrent herpes has already established its pattern, typing is often of little clinical consequence in this setting. Frequent genital herpes recurrences are almost always caused by type 2. If your current or future partner ever wishes to use the Western blot (blood) test for herpes, knowledge of the typing of your virus isolate will be very useful in interpreting the meaning of the result in your relationship.

It is also possible to tell one person's virus from another by its "DNA fingerprint" and thus to trace outbreaks of infection to their source. It seems that the possible variations from strain to strain in this virus are nearly infinite. These tools remain in the hands of researchers for now, although determination of whether your virus is type 1 or type 2 herpes is routinely available.

Herpes Simplex Virus

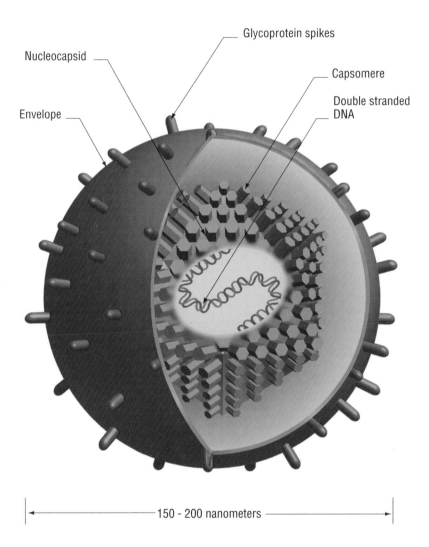

Plate 1: A cross section of herpes simplex virus. The viral DNA is enclosed within a symmetrical icosohedral formation of 192 capsomeres. The lipid envelope contains several types of glycoprotein spikes which are named with letters of the alphabet (e.g., gB, gD, gG, etc.). (p. 31)

Plate 2:

Infection

The DNA of herpes simplex virus is deposited in the nucleus of the infected cell.

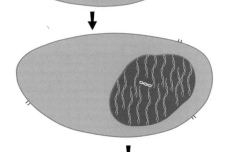

Latency

The viral DNA may remain dormant for an extended period of time directing the production of a few, if any, viral proteins.

Reactivation

The viral DNA "reactivates" and, through the activity of cellular enzymes, begins the processes of replication and synthesis of viral components. Herpes simplex virus produces enzymes such as thymidine kinase and viral DNA polymerase to speed these processes.

(p. 32)

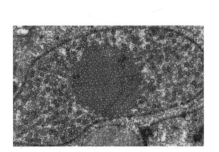

Plate 3: An electron micrograph of the nucleus of an epithelial cell infected with herpes simplex virus. Note the formation and geometric packing of the symmetrical icosohedral nucleocapsids.

96

Color Plates

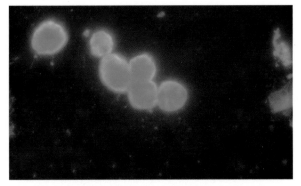

Plate 4: A positive test for herpes simplex virus. Note the apple-green fluorescence at the cell rims resulting from the specific binding of herpes antibody at the membrane. (p. 77)

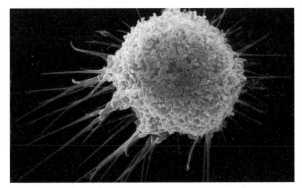

Plate 5: A scanning electron micrograph of a human macrophage. These are the human "janitor" cells. (p. 34)

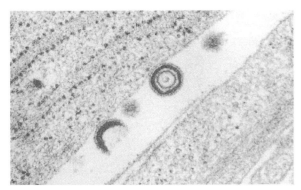

Plate 6: An electron micrograph showing herpes simplex virus sticking to the cell surface.

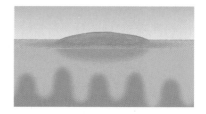

Plate 7a: Early redness/swelling. (p. 52)

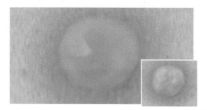
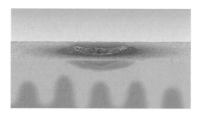

Plate 7b: Vesicle. Inset: inflamed vesicle. (p. 53)

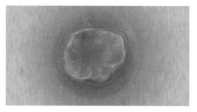
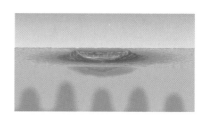

Plate 7c: Ulcer. (p. 54)

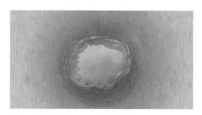
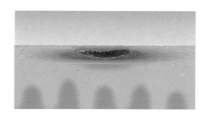

Plate 7d: Wet crust. (p. 54)

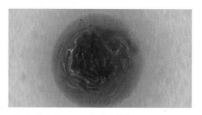

Plate 7e: Dry crust. (p. 54)

Plate 8a: Vesicles clustered on a
swollen red base on thigh. (p. 53)

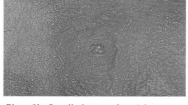

Plate 8b: Small cluster of vesicles on a
swollen red base on penis. (p. 53)

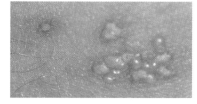

Plate 8c: A classical inflamed vesicular
recurrence. (p. 53)

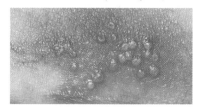

Plate 8d: Inflamed vesicles on penis.
(p. 53)

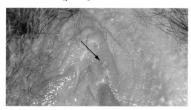

Plate 8e: Wet ulcer on clitoral hood.
(p. 54)

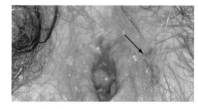

Plate 8f: Wet ulcer on left labium.
(p. 54)

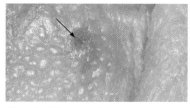

Plate 8g: Wet crusted lesion on penis.
(p. 55)

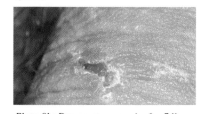

Plate 8h: Dry crust on penis. (p. 54)

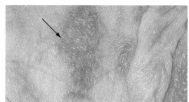

Plate 8i: Residual redness on penis
after healing. (p. 55)

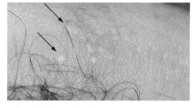

Plate 8j: Residual loss of pigment on
penis after healing. (p. 55)

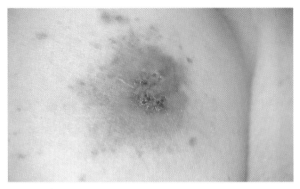

Plate 9: Herpes on buttock. Swelling, vesicles, and crusts are present. (p. 49)

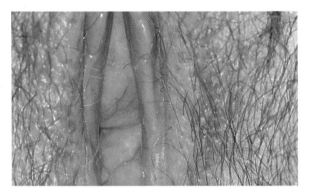

Plate 10: Diffuse redness and irritation of the vulva from a yeast infection (vulvovaginitis). (p. 49)

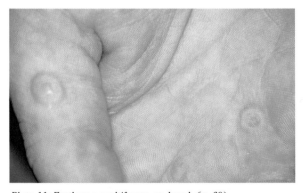

Plate 11: Erythema multiforme on hand. (p. 69)

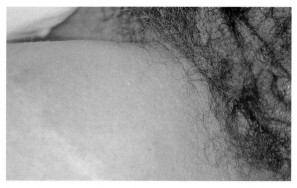

Plate 12: Cellulitis following herpes: note redness and irritation of the vulva and thigh from a streptococcal (bacterial) super-infection. The original herpes lesion is not seen. (p. 69)

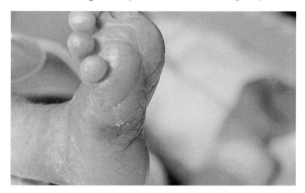

Plate 13: Neonatal herpes on foot. (p. 136)

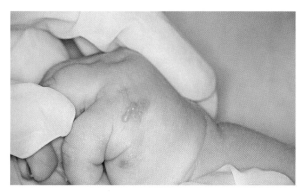

Plate 14: Neonatal herpes on hand. (p. 136)

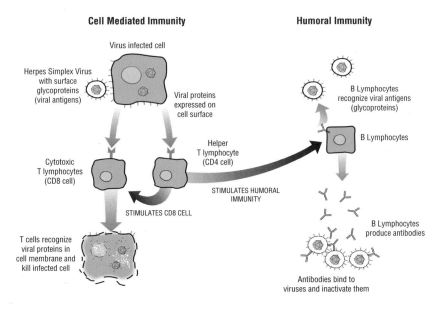

Plate15: The two components of the immune system: cell-mediated and humoral. Each component has a special job in the immune response. (p. 33)

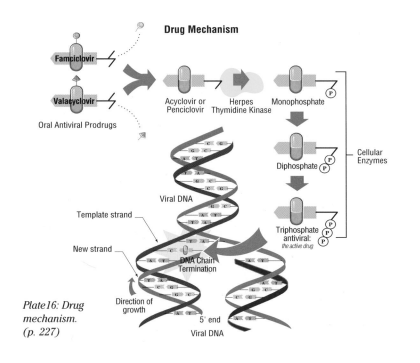

Plate16: Drug mechanism. (p. 227)

5
Genital Herpes: Transmission

Any disease that is treated as a mystery and acutely enough feared will be felt to be morally if not literally contagious.

—Susan Sontag
Illness as Metaphor

How does herpes spread from person to person?

In order to infect a new host, the herpes virus must attach to the epithelial keratinocytes (skin cells). It uses its envelope to hook onto and then fuse together with the membrane of the new cell. Herpes can live only a very short time outside its host cell. Without its surrounding envelope, it dries out and is rendered sterile. Anything that dissolves the envelope, like soap or alcohol, effectively neutralizes the virus. Unlike some other viruses such as the common cold, herpes simplex virus cannot be sent across open spaces (in a room by sneezing, for example), in part because it dries out quickly. (Unlike the daring young man on the flying trapeze, herpes does not fly through the air with the greatest of ease.)

Probably a certain number of virus particles must reach epithelial cells in the new host for infection to be successful. Large numbers are necessary to compensate for the failure of most virus particles to set up effectively in their new host. Similarly, even though pregnancy results from the union of only one sperm and one egg, millions of sperm are required to ensure that one gets through to the egg. How many herpes virus particles are needed for transmission? This is unknown and will probably remain so, since the human experiment required to find the answer is not an ethical one to perform. One can easily imagine, however, that if a very small number of particles were to infect a cell, the reproduction process of the virus might lag behind the immunological defense network within the host. That network is much like an army with specialized units that have a certain starting force. Reinforcements capable of building up each battalion are always on the way. If the invasion force (the virus) is very small, no reinforcements are needed, and the invasion is quashed. If the invasion force is strong, there is a delay until reinforcements come. During the wait for reinforcements, disease occurs. Because of numbers, combined with the fact that the virus loses its ability to cause infection easily when it is outside the body for any significant period of time, direct inoculation is generally required for herpes to spread.

Direct inoculation occurs when infected epithelial cells from one person—preferably kept moist and warm at body temperature and helped by rubbing or, even better, by scratching—come in direct contact with the epithelial cells of another person. Regular skin— on the hand, for example—is protected against all but the most massive invasion because of a natural barrier on the skin called *keratin*. Keratin is waxy and strong. Just as it repels water, it repels herpes virus particles (see figure 1). Unless the keratin is torn, in a cut for instance, the virus cannot get to an epithelial cell. In mucous membranes, however, like those lining the mouth, eye, and genital area, the barrier is very thin, and the epithelial cells are very near the skin surface. This is where access is easiest. On one person, there is an active lesion with herpes growing and alive; add friction for heat and for removal of infected cells from the surface of the donor; add moisture for easy travel and to prevent drying; add exposed epithelial cells of another person; and a new infection is the result.

Thus, genital herpes tends to be sexually transmitted. Other types of transmission are possible but not usual. Most friction, moisture, and heat-producing contact between two people involving the skin of the genitals is sexual. Herpes simplex can be transmitted, for example, from a penile sore to a vagina. However, transmission of genital herpes does not actually require genital penetration. Sexual contact may include a nongenital sore contacting a genital target. In other words, herpes may be transmitted from the source partner's mouth to the other partner's vagina, or from mouth to penis, penis to mouth, finger to penis, penis to anus, or any other combination. The only requirements are infected cells and exposure to new cells belonging to a new, susceptible person, along with heat and moisture. These requirements are also met in a variety of contact sports. Herpes simplex virus does not care if sex is happening. Sure, herpes likes sex, but sex is only one type of contact sport that generates heat, moisture, and friction-based skin-to-skin contact. Herpes can be spread during wrestling, rugby, or any other contact sport that exposes a new susceptible host to infectious virus and thus provides the new environmental opportunities the virus constantly seeks to restart its reproductive cycle in a new host.

What can be done to prevent herpes from spreading?

For herpes to move from one person to another, one person must have herpes and the other person must be susceptible (not have that type of herpes). Further, these two individuals must engage in contact (usually sexual contact) during a period when virus replication is active—growing—on the skin or mucous membrane. When skin herpes is active, protection is achieved by completely avoiding sore-to-skin contact. *A condom does not offer sufficient protection against transmission when a sore is present.*

Anywhere herpes is *active* is a place to avoid having contact. If it is in the mouth, then avoid kissing, oral sex, and so on. If on the finger, keep your hand to yourself while your infection is active. If it is on your thigh, watch what rubs against your partner (try bandaging it). If it is on the genitals, during active infection avoid genital contact and consider using safer (protected) sex practices during other (asymptomatic) times. Using precautions during asymptomatic times will reduce the chance of transmission during those infrequent times when virus reactivates on the skin in very mild episodes. If an active episode is too mild to notice, it is called asymptomatic. The virus is on the skin, just not being noticed.

Herpes generally stays in specific areas of your body. For example, you need not avoid kissing if you have active genital herpes unless you have active sores on your mouth, just as people with cold sores on the mouth needn't avoid genital sex—just putting mouth-to-skin when sores are active. In other words, active herpes is a time to avoid contact with affected areas, but not a time to avoid contact altogether. In fact, it is a time for creative contact. People commonly have sexual contact during which they carefully and successfully avoid putting a finger into their sexual partner's eye. Avoiding sites of active herpes and still having sexual contact is similar. Learn to have contact while avoiding the area of skin actively affected with herpes. This is critical. Total abstinence is okay for a while, but it leads to changes in self-image that are not necessary or useful. They will be discussed later.

You think your active phases are over, but you want to offer your partner maximal protection and want to make absolutely certain that any risk of transmission caused by the small but ever-present chance of asymptomatic shedding is minimized. All people, regardless of herpes history, who have sexual contact without being committed to long-term monogamy are now strongly advised to use condoms. Many physicians also recommend the spermicidal agent *nonoxynol-9*. The latest data on the possibility of asymptomatic transmission of herpes where such protection is lacking make safer sexual practices even more compelling. All people should be taking these precautions unless they are in a monogamous, long-term relationship where the HIV status of both partners is known and there is no ongoing risk of either partner acquiring human immunodeficiency virus from another route. In other words, if one partner in a monogamous sexual relationship continues to share needles with other drug users, his or her sexual partner remains at risk even after a negative blood test. More information on the use of condoms and safer sex techniques is given in chapter 12. During the inactive phases of infection, protected sex using latex condoms will reduce the small risk of transmission and enhance your peace of mind. If your symptoms are over, chances are you've got no virus left on the skin. If you have, chances are it is a small amount. Should asymptomatic shedding occur while you are using condoms properly (see chapter 12), the chances of avoiding transmission are strongly in your favor. A study published in the *Journal of*

Infectious Diseases followed couples over sixteen months where one partner had genital herpes and the other did not (determined by the Western blot test). Asymptomatic transmission did take place in some patients in this study; however, none of the couples in whom asymptomatic transmission took place regularly used safer sex practices.

Some people find that in the beginning—for the first several months after their initial herpes—telling one phase from the next is tricky. Regardless of how you perceive your symptoms, however, in the six months or so following a true primary infection, asymptomatic shedding of herpes is especially common. With careful attention to your body during this period, an awareness generally comes easily. You will get to know your herpes with time. During your getting-to-know period, properly used latex condoms ensure a very low risk of transmission to your partner. If herpes is a new thing in your relationship, however, you will also want to determine with certainty whether your partner has herpes also. If your partner does not have herpes already, then he or she remains at risk of getting it, thus increasing the need for safer sex during the post-primary period. If you have had a true primary infection with type 2 herpes while you were monogamous, however, and you continue to be with the same monogamous partner, there is a reasonable chance that both of you already have genital herpes, regardless of your partner's symptoms or lack thereof. In this case, you would be best advised to determine with your health care provider(s) whether both of you already have herpes. In the meantime, while you are waiting for a reliable answer to this important question, you can always take the position of assuming that your partner is still susceptible to infection. With apologies to Benjamin Franklin, better safe than sorry.

To avoid both herpes and AIDS, careful use of quality latex condoms as a safer sex practice is always recommended. Once both you and your partner understand the risks of getting sexually transmitted diseases (STDs) including AIDS and genital herpes, you can determine how to proceed based on accurate information.

I have herpes on my buttocks (or thigh or foot). How did it get there? Did I spread it from my genitals to this other spot?

This question is an extremely common and important one. If one area on your body can be affected, why not everywhere? Can herpes move around? Herpes sticks to infection of the skin and the local sensory nerves that supply the specific area affected. It does not get tossed around from organ to organ. Herpes is extremely stable in the general area supplied with those nerves. In fact, stability is one of the characteristics that makes herpes so difficult to cure. It gets in one place and sticks with it. There may be a slight variation of the precise skin site from one recurrence to another. This results from the branching of nerve fibers. Herpes strictly follows the nerve to the skin—even if it branches off in a new direction. On one occasion, for example, a herpes reactivation may originate inside one neuron in the ganglion whose nerve fiber supplies a small spot of genital skin of the right side. These nerve fibers have precise routes to the skin and the virus is just as bound to stick with the appointed route as a train is bound to stick to its tracks. It simply cannot veer from its route back to the original skin site any more than electricity can leave the wire on its way from the socket to the lamp, unless a predetermined branch in the tracks or the wire is present.

Therefore, when herpes recurs in a new spot also supplied by the same neural network from the sacral ganglia, you can be certain that the virus did not spill from its tracks. Rather, the reactivating ganglionic cell has a route to the skin that branches elsewhere. This cell could be right next to the cell whose branches go directly to the genitals. In the central switching house of the sacral plexus, cells close enough to be simultaneously infected with latent herpes may lead to related but widely separated areas of skin at the other end of the nerve's branches. Thus, a subsequent "genital" herpes recurrence may find itself in a slightly different area—for example, the buttocks.

Buttock herpes is an interesting and very understudied entity, in general. Probably about 10 percent of people with symptomatic genital herpes get buttock sores sometimes also. Only about 50 percent of people with episodes of buttock herpes are aware of their genital symptoms, but herpes is *almost never* directly inoculated or indirectly autoinoculated to the buttocks. Herpes on the buttocks is a classic demonstration of the nerve branching phenomenon just described. Reactivations emanating from neighboring sacral ganglionic neurons are apparently "wired" to both genital and buttock skin.

So, is buttock herpes the same as genital herpes? Of course, buttocks are not genitals. No, there has not been a recent surge of buttock sex in our society. Nor has there been a new wave of people catching buttock herpes from toilet seats. Buttock herpes is one possible clinical manifestation of genital herpes, because of this nerve tracking business. Many people only get their "genital" herpes on the buttock or thigh or even on the bottom of the foot. As far as we know, people with herpes on the buttock at some point also had genital herpes. That is how the virus got to the neuron that reactivated and branched to the buttock/thigh/foot skin. This may be even more surprising for some people whose lesions feel and look very different when they appear in different spots. So, most sexually transmitted herpes in nongenital skin is not autoinoculated (spread from one part of a person's body to another part) at all. Rather, herpes is following its nerve tracks to alternative routes.

What about true autoinoculation? Can I accidentally spread genital herpes into my eyes? My brain?

People are often concerned about whether they are going to accidentally move this virus all over themselves or to a vital organ by mistake. If, during an active period, you broke a herpes vesicle (blister) with a needle and stuck the needle into your arm, your eye, your lip, or even your brain, for that matter, you probably would develop a new infection at that new site. Injection of herpes from one individual's cold sore into the same individual's arm was actually tested (questionable by today's ethical standards) on prisoner "volunteers" several decades ago. I have had one patient in my clinic who accidentally performed this experiment on himself. He thought that breaking herpes blisters with a needle might help them to heal. (He was mistaken.) Unfortunately, he once slipped and stuck his finger with the needle after breaking his blisters. Now he has herpes recurring on his finger. Aside from such extreme circumstances, however, herpes very rarely winds up moving from one site to another.

Another person I've seen gets recurrent cold sores, usually on the corner of his nose. One August, during an active outbreak, the pollen was heavy in the air. His hay fever was in full bloom along with the flowers. He sneezed and sneezed. He rubbed his itchy eyes and rubbed some more. Later, herpes sores appeared on his eyelids. While this is an example of type 1 autoinoculation, the general principles are the same as for type 2. Extreme circumstances can occasionally result in autoinoculation.

In general, however, autoinoculation is very uncommon after the primary infection is over and the person's immune system has been established against herpes simplex. The immune system prevents most accidental attempts at autoinoculation that might occur from absentmindedness. That does not mean that reasonable personal hygiene is not a good idea. It is only that nature has taken many opportunities to protect us from our own carelessness, making autoinoculation unlikely. During the primary infection, before the immune system is fully established against this virus, autoinoculation is possible. However, the fact that genital herpes is generally held within the confines of underwear means that there is even more protection against this problem.

Autoinoculation to a distant body site (for example, the fingers) is much more likely to occur during the initial attack, especially if it is a true primary. This may occur in up to 10 percent of true primary cases. During this period, immune defenses such as antibodies and lymphocytes are not yet operating at full steam, and therefore little obstruction lies in the path of virus that is anxious to move on to new places using the classical travel characteristics of friction, heat, moisture, and sore-to-skin contact. Immunity will largely prevent the virus from spreading, so, once the primary episode is over, the amount of virus required for new sores to take root is much higher. Immunity alone, however, is not enough of a defense against a lot of virus.

Good hygiene is a good idea. But don't get carried away. Instead of good hygiene, perhaps the word should be reasonable hygiene. Think about what you are doing when you touch your sores. Wash your hands afterwards. Keep contact lenses out of your mouth the same way you should keep them away from your genitals. If sores are active, don't wipe your genitals and then rub your face with the same cloth. Even if you do such a thing, you probably won't have a problem, but why do it? Transmission to your eyes from your own genitals is talked about often but almost never seen. Of several thousand patients I have seen with genital herpes, only two have had type 2 eye infections. Herpes may have been inoculated there at the same time it was inoculated onto the genitals. Auto-inoculation in that situation is unlikely. Genital herpes is not a blinding disease. Herpes of the eye is usually caused by type 1. Generally, that infection is transmitted from the mouth of one person to the face of the susceptible other. Often this occurs from parent to child. The ganglion of facial herpes is called the trigeminal ganglion. The trigeminal nerve supplies sensation to the face through three divisions: mandibular, maxillary, and ophthalmic. The mandibular branch supplies the lower third of the face, the maxillary branch the middle third, and the ophthalmic branch the upper third. Usually, herpes sets up its latent infection in the lower two-thirds—the mandibular or maxillary eye divisions. Cold sores around the mouth are accounted for by those divisions. If, however, the ophthalmic branch of the nerve is infected—e.g., through a kiss to the upper third of the face—then herpes simplex virus will establish latent infection in the ophthalmic division of the trigeminal ganglion. Recurrences from there will follow their appointed "train tracks" and often end up inside the eye. A person can accomplish this with type 2 herpes from the genitals of a partner; it is just a bit more difficult, often involving a slight degree of contortionism. This is not a common clinical problem. Fortunately, ophthalmic (eye) herpes infections in general are getting much easier to treat and suppress with the advent of good antiviral medications.

Genital herpes autoinoculated to the brain is another matter. Rare cases of such events in severely immunologically compromised patients have been reported. Such events are rare even in patients who are severely immunologically compromised. It is safe to say, in general, that encephalitis, or brain infection, is no more likely to happen to the person with genital herpes than it is to anyone else. It is rare, still a bit confusing to scientists as to how and why it happens in the first place, difficult to treat, and extremely dangerous. There is no association at all with genital herpes in adults. Yes, herpes simplex virus type 2 can affect the nervous system. Type 2 herpes can even cause herpes encephalitis, but it does so only extremely rarely in adults. Type 2 herpes of the newborn, however, does cause encephalitis in a small proportion of affected babies (see chapter 6). Frequently, though, type 2 genital herpes causes an inflammation of the protective sac around the brain called the meninges. The inflammation is called *aseptic meningitis* and commonly accompanies a true primary of genital herpes. Meningitis does not damage the brain or you. It can cause a severe headache and/or a stiff neck, however (see chapter 3), and it makes some people temporarily very moody and sensitive to bright lights. Nongenital herpes infections are discussed in chapter 10.

Can I transmit oral herpes to my own genitals?

Could you give yourself genital herpes by rubbing a sore on your mouth and then touching your own genitals? During primary infection in children, this may actually be common. A child with primary oral herpes (usually called gingivostomatitis) who is frequently moving hands from mouth to teething ring to genitalia and back may develop genital sores. These sores are generally type 1 and are seen in the context of a primary facial infection in the child too young to understand disease prevention. Remember, though, this child with primary infection is *nonimmune*. An adult is very unlikely to have this type of problem in this way. The average adult is less likely to get primary mouth infection and is also less frequently going to move his/her hands directly from mouth to genitalia.

Most often when these questions are asked, however, the person has fully recovered from the primary infection and has virtually no problem with autoinoculation. In this case, the immune system is the first protection and is very unlikely to let a second infection through. People who get cold sores often wonder whether they might transmit oral herpes to the genitals of their sexual partner and then become reinfected with their own virus (now their partner's also) back onto their own genitals through genital sex. It is theoretically possible, although extremely rare, for this sequence of events to occur. First, the viral dose required is probably very high. In this case, the person is protected by his or her own immunity against his or her own specific virus. It must be possible, however, for the same reason that the prisoner volunteers described earlier developed sores in the arm. They were immune already, but when enough virus was inoculated by needle into the arm, sores developed. In this case, the transmission method would be sexual, instead. I believe I have seen this occur once or twice in practice, although it must be very rare and difficult to document.

During primary genital herpes, however, autoinoculation is much more readily produced. Local inoculation from one place to another right next to it is normal during the primary. For example, vaginal secretions naturally spread over the perineum, where new sores may develop before your body has developed strong immunity to herpes, which takes a couple of weeks after the first infection starts. Herpes cannot jump from place to place on its own, but if enough virus is put directly into a new place, a new infection may occur.

Can I spread herpes without sexual intercourse—e.g., to my children?

Direct contact is required in order to contract herpes—not necessarily sexual contact. If your child's skin touches your herpes, then of course it can spread. In fact, most herpes simplex virus infections begin during childhood when the baby or child is kissed by a relative or friend with active type 1 herpes on her or his mouth. In general, babies are kissed on the face, but babies may also be (lovingly and appropriately) kissed in all sorts of strange places. I am sure you have seen a doting parent burying their face into the belly button area of a young baby from time to time. Often such strange human activities take place with the expression of unusual and often unrepeatable silly noises from the adult with responsive gurgling, babbling, and laughing from the recipient infant. These "contact sports" keep cropping up all over the place if you really go looking for them.

Objects that pass quickly from one person to another are, theoretically, a possible source of transmission as well. For example, if you share a drinking cup or a cigarette while you have a cold sore, transmission is possible. This is almost certainly a significant source of transmission in families. How about lipstick sharing? You bet. I often wonder how cosmetic counters can allow multiple lipstick testers. Probably, this is not a bigger problem because of the time between customers and whatever little magic the salesperson performs with a cloth. How about bath towels and genital herpes, though? Yes, I would suggest not sharing towels with others while lesions are active. That would logically go for underwear and other intimate articles. I am willing to wager, however, that fewer people share underwear than lipstick. For a lot of reasons not related to herpes, we do not tend to share things quickly from one person to another that involve intimate touching of genital skin in both persons. Furthermore, washing towels and other articles with plain soap dissolves the herpes envelope and kills the virus effectively. There is no need to use special disinfectants or virus killers. I have not seen any good evidence that sharing of bath articles has ever caused one case of herpes. But why risk it? Not sharing bath articles seems a small price to pay! Despite lots of headlines about towels, toilet seats, articles in doctors' offices, and even hot tubs and water slides, no evidence for transmission in these ways has been found. The best evidence is that children are not flocking to physicians with genital herpes. Patients with genital herpes generally avoid giving genital herpes to their children because they do not have sexual contact with their children. It is that simple. That is not to imply that rare exceptions do not exist, because they probably do. You need do no more for prevention, however, than to use reasonable personal hygiene.

What about toilet seats?

The toilet seat argument has been around since toilet seats were invented. Researchers have looked for many diseases, including gonorrhea and syphilis, on toilet seats. Herpes that gets onto a toilet seat, especially a wet, warm one that has not been cleaned in a few days, can stay alive there for quite some time. It does not stay very healthy. It begins to die as soon as it leaves the skin, but it takes a while. If the toilet seat is dried or cleaned, the herpes disappears. If the seat stays wet, the herpes may take an hour or two to fizzle. However, if herpes were alive on the seat, transmission to the next person by this method would still be unlikely, because toileting is not enough of a contact sport. The back of the thigh and the buttocks are thick-skinned areas, relatively resistant to penetration by virus. They are common sites for recurrences, because of the branching of the sensory nerves of the area down to these sites, but the temperature and moisture settings on toilet seats are all wrong for direct transmission to those sites, although nothing is impossible. I have not seen or heard of proven cases of genital herpes from toilet seats or from any other inanimate objects (swimming pools, saunas, water slides). Aside from the lack of friction, moisture, and heat, there are several other reasons which make these sources unlikely. In the case of toilet seats, most public facilities are disinfected regularly with industrial-strength disinfectants that linger on dirty seats and kill germs, herpes included. An experiment suggested that herpes could survive for a few hours on a non-disinfected toilet seat. The authors concluded that maybe toilet seats could serve as a possible source for herpes. However, experiments have never provided any evidence whatsoever for actual transmission by this route. I interpret these findings to show that toilet seats that are not disinfected do not actively kill the virus. Instead, the virus dies slowly on its own. My conclusion from the same data? Do not try to kill your herpes by banging it with a toilet seat, disinfected or otherwise.

I have spent a lot of time on toilet seats in my life and have often wondered how a sexually transmissible virus could get onto the seat in the first place. Certainly if sores are present at the bottom of the buttocks or on the back of the thigh, then those sores will touch the seat. I do recommend that people with sores in those places use toilet paper or seat covers while the sores are in their active phases. They might consider drying off the seat for others, or using a pocket-sized wet napkin. If your sores are on the penis, the labia, the pubic area, or the mouth, the problem is avoided by keeping those areas away from contact with the seat. This seems straightforward to me. The overwhelming majority of people with genital sores never contact the seat with their sores unless they have unusual personal habits. A now late colleague of mine, upon reading in the newspaper about the toilet seat issue, suggested that herpes is transmitted in public toilets only when two people make love in the stall!

No, there should not be separate toilets for people with herpes. My personal bias and infectious disease background suggest that daily disinfection of toilets is a good idea and that toilet seat covers are not a bad commodity. However, these suggestions will help to prevent infectious hepatitis, viral diarrheas, and typhoid fever much more than syphilis or herpes. I remain shocked, as an infectious disease specialist, at how frequently men do not wash their hands after using public facilities. This is the one place in this book where I have limited myself to discussing one gender, since I can honestly say that I do not frequent facilities for women and therefore have no data. We continue to see restaurant-based outbreaks of hepatitis and other bad things that sometimes get into the food from the hands of sloppy cooks. For herpes, though, the toilet seat issue is almost an academic one.

Can I have herpes without having sores?—Asymptomatic shedding

First, the word asymptomatic must be defined. Asymptomatic can mean different things, depending upon the situation. For example, we already know that most people who have genital herpes do not know that fact. These people are all asymptomatic, in the sense that they do not recognize their symptoms and have never realized that they have genital herpes. We also know that if an accurate blood test is used to diagnose herpes in these people (for example, positive type 2 Western blot), and if they are then provided with proper education and counseling and informed of the often subtle and atypical presentations of herpes lesions, then the majority of so-called asymptomatic people with herpes will easily learn within a few months to recognize their symptoms and their active phases of infection.

For people who know about their herpes, however, the issues are different. The question is whether a person can have active herpes virus replication somewhere in or on the genital tract while experiencing nothing at all that suggests an active phase of infection.

This person has had herpes enough times to recognize and understand its active phases and the end of the active phases that comes with the onset of full skin healing. After this point, the chances of recovering virus from the skin through any kind of test are markedly reduced during asymptomatic periods. Asymptomatic shedding (the appearance of virus on the skin without symptoms) occurs on approximately 1 to 5 percent of days, precise results depending on a number of factors that vary from study to study. Several clinical studies have now shown that asymptomatic people with genital herpes who are frequently tested or swabbed for herpes by viral culture during fully healed or asymptomatic phases will have virus on the skin occasionally, when it is not expected. It is entirely normal for this to happen to people with herpes, even people who clearly understand their active phases of infection and people who are being very careful about avoiding sore-to-skin contact during active phases. Presumably, when unexpected virus is found in a study, a very mild episode must be occurring right at that moment that would otherwise go unnoticed.

In many episodes that are thought to be asymptomatic, there are actually symptoms that have not been recognized as herpes. A hemorrhoid that suddenly swells up and itches is usually just a hemorrhoid; occasionally, however, it could be a reactivation of perianal herpes. In fact, studies suggest that asymptomatic herpes is most common in the area around the anus, a very difficult area to see. Intermittent pain in the leg could be a herpes prodrome. An itch in the pubic hair is probably a pimple or just an itch; if there is a little sore behind some hair, however, it could be herpes. The list is endless. This all really means the same old thing: get to know your herpes. Be aware of where your herpes is likely to occur, and avoid contact when an unusual symptom arises there. Wait and see. Do blisters or ulcers (even very small ones) ever develop? If not, your itch is probably just an itch.

The risk of having herpes on the skin when you do not have any symptoms is not great on any specific day, but there is still a definite risk. Dr. Vontver and his coworkers in Seattle studied pregnant women's risk of having a no-symptoms, no-sores, culture-positive recurrence. In the absence of visible lesions, herpes was isolated in 7 of 1,068 cervical cultures (0.66 percent) and 8 of 1,068 external genital cultures (0.75 percent). Another study of pregnant women, by Dr. J. H. Harger and coworkers in Pittsburgh, suggested an asymptomatic rate of virus shedding of about 3 percent. A Vancouver study showed asymptomatic shedding numbers in late pregnancy at about 4 percent. Numbers depend on a number of factors. For example, the immune system may be different in late pregnancy than at other times. Pressure on the vulva from the fetus may alter the rate of recurrences or even make detection more difficult. Yeast infections common in late pregnancy may be easily confused with herpes. In addition, studies vary depending upon how well the subjects undergoing study know the characteristics of their herpes. The sensitivity of the laboratory (how much virus is necessary to get a positive test) may be important, as well as the care of the physician responsible for looking for sores (is this really asymptomatic or missed symptomatic?). In another study, by Dr. S. Straus and his associates from the National Institutes of Health, twenty-six volunteers with frequent genital herpes (but not pregnant or ill in any way) underwent daily genital cultures. Asymptomatic shedding over eleven months occurred in 8 per 1,000 cultures. This accounted for 28 asymptomatic episodes in 26 people, each asymptomatic episode lasting an average of 1.54 days. So asymptomatic genital herpes shedding happens—just not very often and not for very long.

Asymptomatic shedding is more common soon after the primary infection. In fact, for three months after a true primary type 2 infection, cervical asymptomatic shedding is present on about 17 percent of routine visits! Asymptomatic shedding after primary type 1 genital herpes is much lower than after primary type 2. Despite the infrequency and short time span of asymptomatic shedding, recent data suggest that nearly everyone with type 2 herpes has very short, asymptomatic shedding periods every so often.

A recent study by Dr. Anna Wald and her colleagues from the University of Washington followed 110 women very closely for symptoms and viral shedding. This study uses the term "subclinical shedding," defined as all of the active phases of an infection in which a sore is present. Thus, a person who shed virus in this study during a prodromal or warning phase was still identified as subclinical. Over a three-and-a-half-month period, approximately half of the women with type 2 herpes shed virus subclinically. About 29 percent of those with type 1 did so. Women with type 2 herpes shed virus subclinically on approximately 2 percent of the days. The average duration of the shedding period was a day and a half. A common site for subclinical shedding of virus was around the anus. The genital skin, perineum, and cervix were also sites of shedding. In general, the more symptomatic recurrences a woman experienced in this study, the more subclinical recurrences she also experienced. Recent studies show, however, that even people with no history of symptoms of genital herpes will experience subclinical shedding (if they have genital herpes). In fact, it would appear that of the total number of days where virus can be grown from a swab of these areas, about one-third to one-half of those shedding days are identified by the person with herpes as subclinical. This study again showed that the frequency of shedding without signs seemed to decrease somewhat with time. However, this same research group has more recently shown that a person who tends to shed subclinically frequently at one point in time tends to do the same a few years later.

As technology improves, so does our ability to detect herpes when shedding occurs. Over the past few years, Drs. Anna Wald and Larry Corey have aggressively and carefully studied the topic of asymptomatic viral shedding using standard viral cultures, along with a new technique called the *polymerase chain reaction* (PCR). Herpes PCR is so sensitive that it can detect a few molecules of viral hereditary material (DNA) in a swab. (PCR is famous for identification of blood stains during criminal investigations— remember the O. J. Simpson trial?) Using PCR techniques, Drs. Wald and Corey and others have found that herpes DNA can be present in small quantities on the skin far more often than was ever found with viral culture alone. These studies suggest that herpes may reactivate more frequently than has ever been realized before. Apparently, our immune systems are very capable of quickly shutting off herpes when it reactivates. Herpes reactivates from its latent site regularly, but most often the immune response shuts these reactivations off before any living virus makes its way to the skin surface. When the PCR test comes up positive, most of the time there is no surviving virus left—just its PCR fingerprint. The immune system has seen to that. Occasionally, the PCR test and the culture test come up positive at the same time.

PCR may be used as a diagnostic test, because it will not be positive in someone who does not have herpes. When PCR is used to examine for asymptomatic herpes, however, it comes up positive more than 20 percent of the time. What does that mean? The answers are not in yet. While a PCR test cannot be positive in a person without herpes, it can be positive in a person who does have herpes at times where no symptoms are present and no living virus is present on the skin. For now, PCR is an intriguing research tool that will greatly aid in understanding the reactivation process of genital herpes. Since a positive PCR test is common without any living virus, however, it is not entirely clear what it means on a clinical basis. In certain clinical situations, the PCR test has already shown itself to be quite useful for the very reason that it will detect even a remaining fingerprint of the virus. Research in this area will definitely be something to watch carefully.

What are the chances that asymptomatic viral shedding might lead to asymptomatic transmission to my sexual partner?

Two key clinical studies have examined transmission risks in couples. Much more data will become known in the next few years as results from herpes vaccine studies become available. We do know a few key facts. Most people who transmit herpes to their partner do so while they are in an asymptomatic phase of infection. This makes sense, since people do whatever they can to avoid having sexual contact with the affected area while they are in an active phase of infection. Dr. Gregory Mertz and his colleagues followed 144 heterosexual couples for 334 days for evidence of transmission from one person to the other. These investigators were studying a vaccine which turned out to be completely ineffective. The couples were counseled about the active phases of infection and advised to avoid skin-to-skin contact during those phases. They were further advised to use safer sex practices during asymptomatic periods, but only 15 percent of the couples did so regularly. Herpes infections were assessed by the usual methods of diagnosis, including symptoms, cultures, and Western blots. Of 144 sexual partners who were susceptible to herpes, 14 (9.7 percent) acquired infection during this study. In 9 of the 14 cases, no recent symptoms or signs of herpes were reported by the person who transmitted herpes. In 4 of the 14 cases, active phases of infection were reported either during or just after sexual intercourse. In one case, no information was available.

This study showed that the greatest risk for acquiring genital herpes from a partner was based on gender. Women were more than four times as likely as men to acquire genital herpes. In addition to gender, another risk factor was the absence of previous type 1 herpes. More than half of the people in this study (like more than half of the population in general) had antibody to type 1 herpes. People who had no antibody to type 1 herpes acquired genital herpes a little over twice as often as people who had previous type 1 antibody (with or without a history of cold sores). Women who had no antibody to type 1 herpes acquired genital herpes three-and-a-half times more often than women who had type 1 antibody. In this study, couples who regularly used safer sex practices acquired herpes 58 percent less than those who did not. Unfortunately, because so few practiced safer sex regularly, these differences were not found to be statistically significant.

In a separate study from Los Angeles, Dr. Yvonne Bryson studied 57 heterosexual couples where one partner had type 2 genital herpes and the other partner felt that he or she did not. She found that 19 percent of the partners who thought they did not have genital herpes at the start of the study actually did, so they were not counted in the results. The couples were also educated about herpes and about transmission and then followed for approximately 16 months. In this study, the annual rate of transmission (i.e. the proportion of individuals who acquired the herpes virus in one year) to women was 22 percent. For women with no antibody to type 1 herpes, the annual rate was about 32 percent, while it was 16 percent in women who had pre-existing antibody to type 1. Half of the women in this study who acquired type 2 herpes had known, unprotected exposures to active phases of infection in their partners. In this study, none of the men acquired herpes at all. Most of the transmissions occurred early in the relationship, while many couples who had been together for years continued to avoid transmission. Finally, transmission did not occur in any of the couples who regularly used safer sex practices.

These studies demonstrate many important things. First of all, it is impossible in long-term relationships to *completely* eliminate the risk of transmitting genital herpes. While it is not fully proven, there is little doubt that safer sex practices will help to reduce the risks quite substantially. Remember, safer sex practices with herpes means having no skin-to-skin contact with the affected area during the active phases of infection and using condoms properly (see chapter 12) during asymptomatic times. These studies also show that there is reason to hope that a herpes vaccine will someday help to reduce transmission rates, since, in some studies, type 1 herpes antibody itself seems to protect people from getting herpes by at least a factor of two. Furthermore, women are at much higher risk of getting herpes from their male partners than vice versa. Some of the transmissions were avoidable by being careful with active phases, but some were not. It is for those times that safer sex practices can play a very helpful role.

When making choices about preventing herpes transmission, it is clearly wise to consider the possibility that asymptomatic shedding may occur. In case asymptomatic shedding does occur, safer sex practices including proper use of condoms are the best way to minimize the low everyday risk that asymptomatic shedding may lead to asymptomatic transmission. Using sensitive and strict criteria for identifying people acquiring herpes, the University of Washington study showed that simply avoiding sexual contact during the active phases of infection provides enough protection for more than 95 percent of susceptible men and more than 81 percent of susceptible women per year. Both studies clearly showed, however, that simple avoidance during active phases alone is not sufficient to completely prevent transmission. To further minimize the risk of transmission to a susceptible partner, safer sex practices should be used during asymptomatic periods. Be careful, also, about interpreting the word susceptible here. For these studies, susceptible meant that the partner of a person with type 2 genital herpes had no Western blot antibody to type 2 herpes at the beginning of the study period. This is not at all the same as the situation where one person in the relationship has no history of herpes. Western blot antibody to type 2 herpes is present in at least one of five people who have no history of genital herpes. If a person already has Western blot antibody to type 2 herpes, he or she is at minimal risk, from that point on, of acquiring any new type 2 herpes infection from a person with type 2 herpes. He or she may have originally been infected by you or by a different person, depending on the circumstances, but second infections with second strains of type 2 herpes are very uncommon. Second infections are possible, but if a partner who has Western blot antibody to type 2 herpes develops clinical herpes, chances are that any clinical infection in that person will result from their own herpes reactivating.

With all this information about asymptomatic shedding and asymptomatic transmission, what should I do about it?

What have these studies shown us? On the one hand, when looking at the number of days of the year affected, the risk of asymptomatic shedding is really quite low. There is, however, a continuously present, small statistical chance of coming in contact with an active, unsuspected episode of genital herpes. In many long-term partnerships, transmission will not take place even over a period of years. With the passage of time, however, the herpes roulette wheel keeps spinning and small chances build up to significant ones. With each spin of the wheel, the chances remain very low in careful people. Safer sex improves the odds significantly in favor of protection. Don't forget that genital herpes is so common, and so often completely unknown to people who have it, that the everyday roulette wheel of life in the 90s makes the chance of getting herpes from any sexual partner extremely high. It is very common that people who think they do not have herpes actually have it. Type 2 herpes is present in approximately 20 percent of Vancouver women who have had at least one sexual partner and in 55 percent of women who have had at least 10 sexual partners. In the United States, genital herpes may be even more common, with asymptomatic seropositivity rates of up to 30 percent overall in private practice gynecology clinics. Herpes transmission is probably just as likely to occur if one partner thinks he or she does not have herpes and really does have it as it is if he or she knows and is being careful—especially if being careful includes safer sex practices.

In the future, both vaccines and drugs may play an important role in preventing herpes transmission (see chapter 11). Recent studies have also proven that antiviral medications (acyclovir, famciclovir, valacyclovir) taken at least twice daily on a continuous basis (dosing of medicine is something to decide with your doctor) will reduce asymptomatic viral shedding by as much as 75 to 90 percent depending upon the circumstances. Studies are under way to determine if blocking asymptomatic shedding will also block transmission to partners. In general, transmission studies are more difficult to perform. They are very expensive and require the long-term participation of couples in relationships. It is not a big scientific leap, though, to think that if a treatment reduces asymptomatic shedding by 80 percent or more, it might very well reduce transmissions from this shedding as well. If you decide to use treatments to reduce asymptomatic shedding, please note that this is not yet officially approved by regulatory authorities. You should discuss the issues with your doctor carefully before proceeding.

For some partners, the information about risks of transmission is not enough to reassure them. Sometimes, people with herpes worry too much about the potential for transmission. The situation is made worse if the person is very uncomfortable about talking about herpes with partners. A high level of concern and care regarding sexual practices—including limiting the number of partners, using safer sex precautions, and discussing herpes—is now necessary. That is today's reality. *Avoidance of sexual contact altogether because of herpes is not called for under any circumstance.* If you find yourself doing that, however, you are not alone. Many people avoid relationships altogether, in order to keep their herpes secret. Others limit contacts to casual partners in order to avoid discussing it. In either case, the secret itself has become the problem. It is best to begin to undo herpes-caused celibacy as soon as possible. Find a doctor who is comfortable with your problem and who offers specific suggestions for you. If necessary, go for counseling to get your feelings about this sorted out. Share your feelings confidentially with a close friend. Herpes continues to increase in frequency mostly because people are unaware of their infection. You can be very effective at minimizing transmission risk through straightforward rules. It is wise to choose your sexual partner carefully, but staying alone with your secret will not help you or the rest of the world. Approximately 75 percent of all people who have genital herpes do not think they have it and thus, thinking there is no problem, continue to have unprotected sexual contact, with mild sores going unnoticed. Despite all the studies of asymptomatic shedding, the usual source partners of first episodes of genital herpes are people who do not think they have herpes. In other words, the vast majority of partners of people with first episodes of genital herpes are people who thought they did not have genital herpes.

Thus, avoiding sexual contact with a careful person who has herpes may not be an effective means of avoiding this virus. Asking people if they have herpes is also an ineffective test, since most people who have herpes think they don't. A sexual partner who denies having genital herpes could place you at a higher risk of infection than a partner who knows how to avoid transmission of a known and identifiable entity. If your partner has genital herpes and you are susceptible, you are not free of risk, though. You may wish to determine your susceptibility through the Western blot test. If that test shows you to be susceptible, you and your partner are advised to use safer sex practices to decrease the chance of asymptomatic transmission. Stay informed about the availability of vaccines or vaccine studies in your area. Early results from one of the candidate vaccines have been disappointing but additional studies are ongoing. If either you or your partner has a high risk factor for HIV, you may want to get counseling about HIV and be tested for it also, so you and your partner will be in a better position to decide about giving up safer sex practices. If you do not have herpes, though, and you are looking for guarantees that you won't get herpes now or in the future, forget it. The only way to be sure of this is to avoid all sexual contact with all people, regardless of their herpes history, forever.

In summary, regarding the issues of transmission of herpes to a partner, consider the following:

1. Discuss your herpes openly and frankly with your partner before having sexual contact.

2. If your partner has no recollection of having herpes, but has had previous sexual partners, consider asking your health care provider for a Western blot test for your partner to find out whether he or she already has asymptomatic herpes of the same type.

3. Get to know your herpes and avoid all skin-to-skin contact with affected areas during active phases of infection. During active phases you may wish to use sexual techniques that do not include contact with your active areas.

4. Learn about safer sex practices and use them every time you have sexual contact with your partner. After you have all the information and both you and your partner understand the issues, you can decide together about how you want to handle the safer sex issues for the longer term.

5. Discuss with your doctor the possibility of using antiviral suppression to reduce the frequency of asymptomatic shedding, if that appeals to you and your partner. This is not an absolute prevention method, but it does reduce the frequency of shedding substantially. Used in conjunction with the other methods discussed here, it may play a role for you.

6. Find out about the status of vaccinations for herpes. Your doctor or clinic may be participating in clinical trials or know more about one of the new vaccines under study.

If I have herpes, am I immune to a second infection from someone else?

Not fully and completely, but for most practical purposes. A study done in 1980 in Atlanta, Georgia, showed that genital herpes can recur with more than one strain of the virus. People with one strain of herpes can get another. Since immunity is important, it is generally thought that getting herpes a second time is substantially more difficult than getting it the first time. In the section on autoinoculation, a similar question is raised—i.e., can I give herpes to myself in a new place? Transmission of type 2 genital herpes to a person who has Western blot antibody against type 2 herpes is rare. Studies have shown that a person with genital herpes can catch a new case of genital herpes, but other studies have shown that this happens only rarely. In most cases, if a person with genital herpes catches genital herpes while with a partner, they are catching it from themselves (having a recurrence). Type-specific antibody against your own strain of virus makes it very difficult to catch a second infection from a different person.

It takes painstaking effort to tell one herpes strain from another, but it can be done. The test is not one a family doctor or even a specialist can perform. In order to tell the herpes of Mr. Jones from the herpes of Ms. Smith, a "DNA fingerprint" is obtained: the virus is grown in the laboratory and purified, and the DNA (see chapter 1) is extracted with chemicals. Then, enzymes called restriction endonucleases are added, which cut the DNA in several special places. The small pieces that are left are put into a wobbly but firm gel and an electric charge is introduced, causing the pieces to travel inside the gel. This test bears some similarity to the Western blot test, in which small proteins travel inside a gel. In this case, the travelers are small pieces of DNA. Since small pieces travel faster than large ones, the gel makes a "fingerprint." Using this method, researchers have shown subtle differences between the fingerprints of different virus strains. Rarely, two strains on separate recurrences in the same person and dual infections of two strains at the same time have been observed. However, second infections with new strains are considered to be extremely rare. Studies that have sought different strains from a single person with genital herpes have had a very difficult time finding them in most people. Yet statistics suggest that people with genital herpes commonly come in contact with herpes more than from more than one partner. There must be a very strong immunity to second infection, although it is not yet defined scientifically. Although incomplete, immunity to type 1 herpes affords a very high degree of protection against infection with type 2 herpes. This protection makes type 2 somewhat more difficult to get. Antibody to type 1 herpes, however, does not *fully* protect against type 2. Many people who get type 2 herpes do so despite having this type 1 partial protection. People with type 1 who do get type 2 will, by definition, not experience a true primary. The first episode will likely be less severe than for people who have no preexisting immunity to type 1 or type 2. It may be that people with type 1 immunity are somewhat predisposed to acquire type 2 genital herpes asymptomatically, should they come in contact with type 2 herpes and acquire infection from a partner. Since their bodies are already fully equipped to fight off the infection effectively, people with type 1 herpes are probably more likely not to notice infection with type 2. Type 1 herpes is just as likely as type 2 herpes, however, to be acquired without any evident symptoms—so, while a history of recurrent oral cold sores is strongly suggestive of type 1 herpes simplex, the absence of such a history provides absolutely no evidence that a person does not have latent herpes simplex virus type 1. Only type-specific antibody tests like the Western blot are able to do that.

How could this happen to me?

Herpes infection can happen to anyone. Several careful epidemiological studies have proven this. Approximately four out of five people with genital herpes acquire their genital herpes infection some time between their eighteenth and thirty-sixth birthdays. The overall incidence of genital herpes (apparent and unapparent) is increasing constantly. Most genital herpes infections are unknown to the people who have them (asymptomatic or unapparent). The group of people at greatest risk are women between the ages of twenty and twenty-four. Depending upon the group being studied, approximately 16 to 33 percent of Americans have antibody to type 2 herpes simplex virus. In other words, those people actually have type 2 genital herpes, even though most of them do not recognize that fact. On a statistical basis, the more sexual partners a person has had, the more likely that he or she will have antibody to type 2 herpes. In all age groups, African-Americans have been shown to be at greater risk of having antibody to type 2 herpes than Caucasians of the same age. Australians have about half to two-thirds the incidence of type 2 herpes compared with North Americans. Observations regarding income of people with herpes have been somewhat inconsistent. In many studies, antibody to type 2 herpes is more prevalent in people of lower income. However, in one Stanford study, Hispanic women who were of upper middle class income were far more likely than lower income women to be seropositive for type 2 herpes (30 percent versus 17 percent). Studies from herpes self-help groups also show very high levels of education and income among people diagnosed with herpes. I am sure that it is not the college or the job that gave that person genital herpes. Nor is herpes caused by a specific race or socioeconomic class.

Herpes literally knows no boundaries. Even sexual habits may not correlate in any one individual to the acquisition of infection. You only need to have one lifetime sexual partner to get genital herpes. Even if both you and your partner have only been with each other in your whole lives, it is quite possible for you to get type 1 genital herpes from oral-genital sexual contact if your partner has mouth infection. If your partner has had previous sexual partners even a long time ago, there is a good chance that he or she has come across this infection. If your partner has had more than ten sexual partners in the past, he or she is statistically likely to have been infected with herpes. By statistical chances alone, people with more sexual contacts are more likely to acquire this virus. There is an additional approximately 5 to 6 percent risk for each additional sexual partner. However, herpes has become so universal that many people who have had only one or two sexual contacts have herpes. Since genital herpes is predominantly an external disease, sexual contact that results in transmission does not necessarily include vaginal penetration. Several well-documented cases of herpes in women who have not had vaginal intercourse have been described, almost always the result of oral-genital contact.

As a society, we have subjected ourselves to a higher chance of running into herpes, partly by giving up condoms and foam for the convenience of the intrauterine device (IUD) and the pill and partly because sex has become less forbidden. Oral sex has become commonplace, while oral-to-oral transmission of type 1 herpes simplex virus in childhood has become less likely. These factors lead to an increase in oral-to-genital transmission of herpes. Herpes infection of some type is found in most people on earth. Sores on the genitals usually come with more emotional baggage than sores on the mouth. But the stigma attached to genital herpes is mainly a media phenomenon. Genital herpes is basically a nuisance skin infection that comes and goes. It has unusual complications that are unlikely to occur and are highly preventable.

Some people have suggested that the growing incidence of herpes is a new demonstration of the wrath of God. In response to this, I would point out that elimination of all but monogamous sexual contact would cut down the overall incidence of this infection, but monogamy would not eliminate herpes. A person who was monogamous or even sexually inactive could get genital herpes. Increasing the numbers of sexual partners statistically increases the chances of getting any sexually transmitted disease. For the sake of prevention of disease, it is and always has been wise to be selective, to know your partner, to avoid casual sex, etc. Religious preference does not correlate in any way to susceptibility to infection, however. Herpes is no more a sign of punishment from God than Legionnaire's disease was a sign of punishment from God inflicted upon the American Legion. Ascribing any new disease or affliction, or any old disease or affliction, to the plagues of God is rewriting the Bible. In the case of herpes, it is also the result of misinformation.

I had sex last night and awoke with a sore. Did I spread herpes to my partner? Should my partner be taking an oral antiviral drug to prevent infection?

Probably not, if you had no symptoms of active infection when you had genital contact. Herpes shedding does not generally begin before the symptoms of an outbreak, although studies done at the University of Washington did show that shedding of virus just before the onset of genital symptoms was the probable source of asymptomatic transmission in several cases. In some cases, a recurrent herpes sore will start out as an asymptomatic episode, probably because the sore is too small or mild to detect. For whatever reason, it goes unnoticed. Then, by the next day, the sore is bigger or more swollen or more uncomfortable—in other words, more symptomatic. This is not the normal situation, but it is apparently not rare either. To awaken with a sore without having had or having noticed a prodrome is a relatively frequent event that is usually, although not always, a new event, totally unconnected to the asymptomatic day or night before.

Furthermore, if sexual contact is a daily occurrence, then every time you awake with herpes you will have had sex the night before. If you have followed the guidelines for preventing transmission, including use of safer sex practices, then even if you had a small sore that went unnoticed, your partner will have been protected by those just-in-case efforts. However, if you think that you may have exposed your partner to direct contact with an active sore, then your partner may wish to consider using one of the oral antiviral drugs, because even though this type of treatment is unproven for this purpose, there is every reason to believe that it could provide some protection following exposure in some people (see chapter 11). This is not a method to count on, however. As a side note, there is no scientific justification for a susceptible partner to take antiviral medications on a long-term or continuing basis. Preventive use for one week after a likely exposure is also unproven but makes some sense based on research in animals and on the high degree of safety seen with these medicines. Long-term use by someone who does not have herpes at all would be quite another matter. For further information, refer to chapter 11.

Can I have a long-term relationship with one person and never transmit herpes?

Yes, such relationships are very common. Dr. Charles Prober at Stanford University has found that couples are very commonly "discordant"—that is, one person has type 2 genital herpes—without transmitting it to the partner, often for a very long time.

In general, the chance of not seeing an active sore becomes higher as the number of encounters between two people increases. It is often the case, however, that when herpes is transmitted after a couple has been together for several years with only one partner affected, there has been an event during which the barrier to active infection broke down. A break in the barrier to active infection can occur because of a mistake, because of a choice, or because of asymptomatic virus shedding.

In time, many couples lose their desire to hold to strict rules to avoid transmission. Since herpes is usually physically mild, some people in permanent relationships decide that prevention is not worthwhile. Once the issue of discussing herpes with your partner has been dealt with and the relationship has established itself as long-term, couples often choose to ignore the small ongoing risk of transmission and begin taking risks.

Speaking of risks, we take them all the time. We risk our lives driving in cars; we risk our genital health having sex. To take risks is human. To take risks with someone with herpes is also human and, relative to some other risks, not so big. Deciding which risks are right for you is up to each individual and each couple.

6
Herpes of
the Newborn

*Every mother entertains the idea that her child will be a
hero, thus showing her wonderment at the thought of
engendering a being with consciousness and freedom; but
she is also in dread of giving birth to a defective or a
monster, because she is aware to what a frightening extent
the welfare of the flesh is contingent upon circumstances-
and this embryo dwelling within her is only flesh.*

—SIMONE DE BEAUVOIR
The Second Sex

What is herpes of the newborn?

Despite dramatic breakthroughs in knowledge, our understanding
of immunology (the body's defense network) leaves a lot unexplained. The immunology of the newborn baby is especially confusing. At birth, many changes take place. The heart begins
pumping blood in a different direction, the lungs inflate with air for
the first time, and the baby becomes a free-living organism facing
the external environment. Most babies thrive in this new environment. For reasons that are only partially understood, some babies
are highly susceptible to infection.

Many different infectious agents cause infections in newborns
under certain circumstances. Most of these agents are entirely tol-
erable to adults. They may even be normal flora—a part of the normal (indeed, necessary) colony of bacteria or fungi that cause
absolutely no disease in adults. One example of normal flora is the
bacteria *Escherichia coli*, which inhabits the gut of nearly everyone. Commonly, a woman gets some of these bacteria into her
bladder—often as a consequence of minor trauma from sexual
contact—and a urinary tract infection (cystitis) results.

Most babies tolerate this organism. Essentially all babies are
exposed to it during birth. Of 1,000 babies who are exposed, 998

could not care less. However, an unfortunate one or two of the thousand develop severe, overwhelming infection—even meningitis—and may suffer severe damage or even die. In some of these babies, the reason for infection is obvious—for example, prolonged rupture of the membranes, where exposure to bacteria may be very intense and sustained over a long period. In other cases, the reasons for infection remain unknown.

Why should a newborn baby be so susceptible to infection? Every baby's immune system is somewhat immature. Immune experience is nearly as undeveloped as job experience at birth, except that the mother's blood gives some immune experience to the baby by passing along antibodies, which filter across the placenta. Newborns are born possessing many of the same antibodies as their mothers. While inside the uterus, the fetus is protected from most infection by the filtering capabilities of the placenta, which excludes almost all infecting agents; at the time of birth, the newborn has not yet had to respond to infection. All those lymphocytes and macrophages and so forth, which do most of the immune fighting against foreign invaders, have never been stimulated before. Just as the newborn has never before seen the light of day, so her or his white blood cells have never seen a bacterium. The cells are just beginning to learn how the system works. Thus, occasionally, a baby succumbs to an infection that would cause only a mild illness or no problem at all in you or me.

Herpes of the newborn is one example of this problem. Herpes simplex, which causes a mild skin infection in the adult, may, under certain circumstances, overcome the immature immune system of a newborn baby and disseminate throughout the body, resulting in death, or ascend up the immature nervous system into the brain, resulting in encephalitis with consequent brain damage, or invade the eye, resulting in eye infection and eye damage. Such complications are very unlikely to occur in any individual newborn. All studies in the past decade have shown that herpes simplex infection is extremely unlikely to occur to any one individual baby born to a woman with genital herpes. In fact, the woman's infection with herpes before pregnancy even offers some protection to the baby if exposure to active herpes takes place. Curiously, more than half the babies born with herpes have mothers who did not know they had herpes. If a pregnant woman knows she has genital herpes, newborn herpes is largely preventable and highly unlikely. Herpes is not a reason to avoid having children, because the baby of a woman with genital herpes is extremely unlikely to have any problems with neonatal (newborn) infection.

What are the signs?

Just as the symptoms of genital herpes vary with the location of the infection, so do the signs of neonatal herpes. In some unusual cases, herpes is already present at birth. Since infection usually begins at the time of birth, however, it most commonly takes several days to a couple of weeks to become evident. The most common herpes infection in newborns is on the skin. The skin sore looks much like a sore on an adult—i.e., a single vesicle (blister) or cluster of vesicles. Occasionally, herpes begins as a red or purplish rash. Because many very mild skin rashes of infancy mimic herpes, it is important to ask a doctor's opinion when a skin rash develops in a newborn—especially if a sore similar to those pictured in chapter 3 develops. Almost every baby has some type of skin rash at some point in the first few weeks of life. Normal things called *milia*, for example, which look like little pimples, may be frightening to the mother with genital herpes who thinks her baby has the infection. Milia are very, very common; several babies in every nursery have them. Expect to see a skin rash on your baby just because he or she is a baby. Genuine herpes sores may be found anywhere on the skin, especially on the head of a baby born head first, the buttocks of a baby born rear first, and so on. Plate 13 (page 101) shows a newborn who was delivered feet first. Skin lesions in a newborn are not always or exclusively at the site of the presenting part, however. Plate 14 (page 101) shows the recurrent herpes on the hand of a baby that had neonatal herpes at birth.

Another common site of herpes of the newborn is the eyes. Most babies have red and swollen eyes because of the silver nitrate put in their eyes at birth to prevent infection. Generally, the redness and discharge fades quickly over the first few days of life. Herpes in the eye most often appears as redness—*conjunc-*

tivitis—with or without discharge of pus from the eye. Herpes infection of the eye is often detectable only by an examination by an ophthalmologist (eye specialist).

Most studies suggest that many newborns who develop genital herpes never develop skin lesions at all. The more severe neonatal herpes syndromes are infection of the central nervous system (the brain) and infection that disseminates through being carried in the blood and distributed in many parts of the body. Brain infection tends to appear at one to four weeks of age. An affected baby may suddenly lose his or her active behavior and become lethargic. The baby may stop caring about things such as feeding, or may do just the opposite and become very irritable. This, of course, is a very common thing in normal babies as well, but an irritable baby should be assessed to make sure it is nothing more than "just colic." Shaking, twitching, or fits (like epileptic fits) should be checked out by a physician without delay. Babies with herpes infection of the nervous system may have skin sores, but very often a baby with serious herpes infection shows no skin problem whatsoever.

The same is true for disseminated herpes; skin sores may or may not be present. Dissemination appears a bit earlier, often within the first seven days of life. In most cases, herpes is present at birth, implying that herpes infected the baby inside the womb. There is no known specific method for prevention of womb infection. Most babies with dissemination have nonspecific symptoms, including lethargy, going off feeding, and vomiting. An affected baby may become gravely ill very rapidly. *Jaundice* (yellow skin) is very common in infants. When associated with actual liver enlargement and abnormal blood tests of liver function, jaundice may be the result of herpes or it may be caused by many other things. Sometimes a baby with herpes gets *pneumonia*, has difficulty breathing, or has *apnea* (spells with no breathing at all). These are serious problems that require intensive investigation in hospital. If the mother has herpes, the pediatrician needs to know in order to consider this possibility.

All of the scenarios discussed above, with the possible exception of skin sores, have nonspecific symptoms. This is the problem. So many things—some infectious, some noninfectious; some very serious, some very minor—present themselves in exactly the same way. Reading this section may be frightening, but reading the list of symptoms of any disease can be frightening. Even if your baby gets all of these symptoms, herpes is unlikely. Neonatal herpes is exceedingly unlikely to occur and is highly preventable. Furthermore, if it happens in spite of efforts at prevention, it is treatable. In fact, the problem with treatment is less the difficulty of finding a useful drug and more the delay that often occurs before the diagnosis is made. If the first sign of something serious is nonspecific, it may take days to find the correct diagnosis. The delay makes treatment more difficult. If your infant becomes ill, get medical attention. Herpes can be diagnosed only if it is looked for; tell your physician about your herpes to make sure he or she considers herpes as a possibility. You should not attempt to make your own diagnosis.

Is direct contact during delivery the only way of giving herpes to a baby?

No, but it is by far the most common way of transmitting it. Most often, newborn herpes infection results from a lack of awareness by everyone concerned. Most people (including pregnant women) with herpes never know that they have herpes. Once recurrent herpes has occurred, nature takes over and, by a series of brilliant maneuvers, effectively prevent herpes transmission to the newborn in the vast majority of potential cases. Once recurrent herpes has been diagnosed, the woman and her health care provider can do many more things to prevent transmission. We are learning, however, that we have to be careful in trying to improve on the prevention techniques of nature, because some of our previously accepted prevention techniques have proven to be worse for the mother than the very low risk of neonatal herpes ever was. Babies of women with recurrent genital herpes are largely protected from infection with herpes, for reasons described later in this chapter.

When herpes is not diagnosed before the woman gives birth, however, prevention is left entirely up to nature. In the case of recurrent herpes, the baby may be exposed to active virus on the mother's skin. This does not lead to any problem in the newborn in the vast majority of cases, but physicians generally believe that if exposure to known virus on the skin in an active phase of infection can be prevented during labor and delivery, it should be. In other words, someone who is having an active recurrence should have a cesarean section. There is argument about this, too, however, since there is a small but significant risk of complications from cesarean section. In most cases, a baby born to a mother having an active herpes episode will not develop any disease as a result of this exposure, so we should be very careful in trying to improve on this already impressive capability of nature.

The situation is different, however, if a woman develops primary herpes or nonprimary type 2 herpes (first time ever in a patient who has never been previously exposed) during the last few days or weeks of pregnancy. It is common for first episodes of infection to begin with nonspecific symptoms—for example, vaginal discharge, fever, or urinary discomfort. There may not be obvious external sores early on. The woman experiencing a first episode may very well not realize what is going on and therefore not warn her physician. Furthermore, a visual search for herpes may not be done during labor and delivery. The exam for herpes is a visual one and includes a search for uncomfortable sores on the vaginal lips, on the perineum, around the anus, under the pubic hair, and on the cervix. The usual obstetric exam during labor, however, is a manual one—a search for the progress of labor, using the fingers to feel the cervix. Feeling with the fingers does not detect herpes sores. The eyes detect herpes. Newborns of mothers having a first episode herpes infection are likely to be undiagnosed and are also especially susceptible to getting herpes.

So what should be done to prevent transmission of herpes to the newborn? People must learn to think about herpes when vaginal discomfort or other symptoms appear during the latter part of pregnancy. Physicians who deliver babies must make their eyes an important part of their medical tool kits during labor. Every woman in labor, regardless of her history, should be assessed for herpes by careful examination. Some hospitals have begun to assess each woman by virus culture as well, but, because results take one to several days to be returned, viral culture cannot be used to determine whether cesarean section is necessary. If active genital herpes is visible near the birth canal, cesarean section is probably advised, even for a woman with recurrent genital herpes. However, if no lesion is present, the very low risk of transmission of herpes does not warrant the use of cesarean section for the prevention of herpes. In contrast, where a first episode (primary or nonprimary) of genital herpes occurs in the late second or third trimester of pregnancy, neonatal herpes risk can be greater. In such situations, some specialists would recommend treatment with acyclovir for ten days, even though no studies have been performed and no clear guidelines are available. Some (but not all) would restart acyclovir for the last four weeks of pregnancy. For now, this is an individual decision and must be made between the woman and her physician.

Neonatal herpes can occasionally be caused by infection after birth. These cases are relatively unusual. Since the mother may not even have herpes, there is a high chance that the baby will be born without immunity from the mother and be very susceptible. Exposure can come, for example, from the kiss of a parent or nursery attendant who has an active cold sore. The *herpetic whitlow* (herpes of the finger) is an especially important cause for concern, since this infection is often misdiagnosed (see figure 11, page 199). Because the herpes is on the finger, any finger-to-skin contact from the affected person when whitlows are active could result in transmission of herpes. Also, if another baby in the nursery has herpes, a nurse who handles the infected baby and does not wash his or her hands might pass on the virus to another infant. Happily, hospitals have strong infection control measures to prevent this.

Infection can also occur inside the womb, although this occurs rarely. Probably most fetuses infected with herpes early in gestation (their time inside the womb) do not survive and are miscarried. Because infection with herpes can be spotty, however, it is possible for infection to occur at one area that is not crucial to survival and for the fetus to develop in spite of this infection. Near term, it is possible (though unlikely) for little holes in the amnion (sac of waters) to open and reseal, allowing infection in. Fortunately, this is unlikely to lead to herpes infection. Herpes infection in the newborn generally occurs during birth. The congenital (inside the womb) herpes syndrome does exist, however, and there is nothing that can be done specifically to prevent it. It cannot be predicted on the basis of the type of infection or by special tests. There is no greater risk in babies whose mothers have five outbreaks per month than in those whose mothers have one outbreak per year. In fact, why it ever happens is poorly understood. Some cases result from true primary herpes during pregnancy.

Can I transmit herpes by kissing my baby?

Yes, as described above. Neonatal herpes can be type 1 or type 2. Approximately one-fourth of neonatal infections are type 1. It is not actually *proven* that kissing is an important source for neonatal herpes. It is likely that type 1 neonatal herpes often results from the mother's primary genital type 1 infection. It is prudent to assume that kissing and other nongenital contact can also cause neonatal herpes, despite academic argument to the contrary. A kiss from a herpes-infected mouth can transmit herpes as well as a delivery through a herpes-infected vagina. If you have sores on your mouth just after the baby is born, transmission must be carefully avoided. (Of course, people with genital herpes do not have to avoid kissing newborns. Genital herpes cannot jump from your genitals to your mouth to your baby.)

What is done to prevent transmission after birth? First, if herpes is not active in the mother, nothing special is done. Birth proceeds normally and the baby is treated exactly like any other baby. He or she may room in, or stay in the nursery, or both. Whatever you want to arrange with the doctor and the hospital is just fine. If herpes is *active* on the genitals when labor begins, a cesarean section is performed (more on that later), and the baby should usually room in with the mother or be in a special area of the nursery. Otherwise, things are routine. You need not wear a mask unless you have a sore on your mouth. You need not wear gloves unless you have a sore on your hands. You can breast-feed without problems unless you have a sore on your breast. You should not find yourself in strict isolation in the hospital because of herpes. You might find an isolation sign on your door saying "Contact Isolation" or "Wound and Skin Isolation", meaning that your sore, if active,

141

should be isolated while you are in the hospital. Nothing else need be isolated. Most precautions in hospitals make sense. Someone should be able to explain why you and your baby need or do not need to be isolated. There should be neither too little nor too much isolation. If your questions are not properly answered, you might ask to speak with the infection control officer (usually a nurse or physician) for an explanation.

Why does first episode primary or nonprimary type 2 herpes during pregnancy pose a much greater risk for the newborn?

Primary herpes affects the mother's whole body. Illness in the mother can cause early labor and premature birth, a significant risk factor for developing neonatal herpes. Primary herpes occurs, by definition, before the mother has acquired any immunity to herpes. Nonprimary type 2 first episodes of herpes occur before the mother has acquired any immunity to that virus. As the mother has no immunity to pass on to the baby, the baby is born susceptible to herpes infection. Furthermore, because primary herpes in most cases involves the internal parts of the birth canal, including the cervix, exposure of the newborn is much more likely to occur. First episodes of herpes are very likely to go undiagnosed because the symptoms are often nonspecific and the diagnosis unsuspected. In addition, the amount of virus shedding is very high compared with a recurrent episode—as much as a thousand times more. Viral shedding tends to last for ten to fourteen days, rather than two or three days in a recurrent episode.

What if my partner has genital herpes and I do not?

Some studies have suggested that we may be better able to prevent neonatal herpes in the future by focusing more on undiagnosed cases of maternal primary infection. The best way to prevent primary or nonprimary type 2 herpes infections in pregnant women is to prevent exposure to herpes during pregnancy. One logical way to do this is to identify situations where the pregnant woman's sexual partner has genital herpes and the pregnant woman does not. Dr. Charles Prober and his colleagues at Stanford University have begun to study the possibility of identifying such *discordant pairs*, in which the partner has herpes and the pregnant woman does not. That combination has the potential for a bad outcome. People who have herpes should discuss this with their partners if pregnancy is planned. The pregnant woman who has never had herpes and who continues to have sexual contact with a partner with herpes is in a powder keg situation, as far as neonatal herpes is concerned. It is important that she not acquire infection for the first time during pregnancy, especially toward the last trimester. If she gets herpes before pregnancy, then the baby is at low risk because of the reasons given elsewhere in this chapter. If she gets herpes after pregnancy, the baby is not, of course, at risk. However if she gets herpes for the first time during pregnancy, the baby's risk is significant. Accurate determination of her susceptibility requires the type-specific blood test, as outlined in chapter 4. Couples who have given up safer sexual practices should readopt them during pregnancy if the pregnant woman remains susceptible to herpes. Safer sex in this case means avoiding genital sexual contact altogether during active phases of infection and using the prevention techniques described in chapter 12 when having sexual contact at inactive times. The couple should take every possible measure to prevent transmission of herpes during the pregnancy.

Preventing transmission of herpes during pregnancy will be one of the most important challenges for any new herpes vaccine. You can read more about vaccines in chapter 11.

If a pregnant woman does acquire true primary genital herpes, I advise the following:

1. Document the infection, using viral culture of the lesions.

2. Rule out other sexually transmitted diseases and the common vaginal infection bacterial vaginosis, since they can also have special impact during pregnancy, if left untreated.

3. Determine whether it is a primary or nonprimary type 2 herpes infection. This is possible in most cases by determining that the initial serology (Western blot) test for herpes is totally negative (true primary) or negative for type 2 and positive for type 1 (nonprimary), meaning that the person is susceptible. If this negative test is combined with a positive viral test for herpes

from the genital tract, the diagnosis of a true primary or a non-primary genital herpes infection is confirmed.

4. If a primary is suspected during a first episode, because of severe lesions on both sides of the body, fever, cervical involvement, inguinal lymph node (gland) swelling and tenderness, or urinary symptoms, or, if a possible primary infection is documented (as discussed above), then systemic treatment with acyclovir may be warranted, despite the fact that the safety of acyclovir during pregnancy is not fully proven (see below).

5. In some situations, your doctor may decide with you to prescribe oral acyclovir for treating your first episode. However, this is an individual clinical decision between you and your doctor, since no scientific studies are available to provide guidelines.

6. You and your doctor should discuss the option of cesarean section if your primary or nonprimary first episode of genital herpes infection took place during the third trimester of pregnancy, regardless of the clinical state of your herpes at the time of labor. This is not a proven approach and has not been discussed much in the medical literature. However, the risk of having a positive cervical culture in the absence of any symptoms is higher than usual during the first three months after the primary. This risk, which is much higher than the risk of asymptomatic shedding during any later asymptomatic phase of genital herpes, may warrant planned cesarean section (at term) for a woman who has had a first genital infection in the third trimester. Cesarean section for asymptomatic herpes is not warranted in any situation other than the true primary or nonprimary first episode in the third trimester, however, for reasons outlined elsewhere in this chapter.

Why am I advised to avoid acyclovir during pregnancy, on the one hand, and to use acyclovir during pregnancy, on the other hand?

There is every reason to believe that the use of acyclovir during pregnancy is *probably* safe. Probably safe is not good enough, of course, to warrant the use of this drug for trivial reasons. Therefore, in most cases where it does not matter, acyclovir should be discontinued during pregnancy. This is especially important during early pregnancy, when the risk of harm to the fetus is greatest. In the third trimester, the fetus has formed most of its key organs already. Acyclovir does not *seem* harmful, so far, even where it has been used in early pregnancy. Studies have shown that untreated primary herpes in the third trimester may result in a significant medical problem for the newborn in up to 50 percent of cases. Therefore, intervention with treatment is very logical. Treatment of the pregnant woman with acyclovir, however, has not been fully *proven* to be safe or effective. Although there is no scientific evidence, it is possible that there could be a benefit to the woman and the fetus by reducing the severity of primary herpes, including the viral load and the duration of complications, which could theoretically reduce the chance of the baby developing a medical problem.

This opinion is guesswork, though, in the absence of a study. Some doctors and scientists argue that it is better to let the mother acquire the best possible immunity to the virus on her own. Treatment with acyclovir probably limits the degree of immunity the mother acquires, by limiting the amount of time and the degree to which she is exposed to the virus in order to develop immunity to it. In theory, that could wind up being worse for the baby than no treatment at all. I believe it is important to limit the severity of the primary episode, if at all possible. But this course of action is unproven and should be decided in each individual case by the woman and her doctor. No one simple answer is available now, and the chance of a definitive clinical trial is minimal. Chances are we will continue to do what we think best. The more acyclovir's safety record suggests that it is free of significant harm in pregnancy, the better this approach appears.

What about the newer antiviral drugs, famciclovir and valacyclovir?

Both are probably safe in pregnancy, but because there is far less clinical experience with new drugs, acyclovir should probably be the main drug to consider when using a drug in pregnancy. You will have to make this decision with your doctor, however, and he or she is the best source for up-to-date information about risks and benefits.

If I get primary herpes during early pregnancy, should I have an abortion?

If herpes were ever to spread into the womb, it would be most likly to occur during primary herpes, before immunity to the virus is established. If a fetus were to be infected with herpes early in gestation, the likelihood of miscarriage would probably be very high. A recent study by Dr. Z. A. Brown from the University of Washington described the outcome of fifteen cases of primary genital herpes during pregnancy. One of the five fetuses of women affected during the first trimester (twelve weeks) was spontaneously miscarried and had been infected in the womb with herpes. The other four were fine. Subsequent studies by Brown have suggested that the actual risk to the fetus of primary infection in the first trimester may be much smaller than the small initial studies suggested. But more work needs to be done.

Is herpes, then, an indication for therapeutic abortion? A lot will depend on the woman's attitude toward abortion and toward the pregnancy. Even if a woman is in her eighth week and having full-blown primary herpes, her fetus's risk of becoming infected in the womb is low. Exactly how low remains to be determined. The woman must decide what to do. By no stretch of the imagination is genital herpes a necessary reason to have an abortion.

In order to make any decision about a possible abortion, or any other course of action, you must first be certain you have your facts straight. Recurrent herpes and nonprimary first episodes are not reasons for abortion, so you should be quite certain first that what you had was a true primary. Clinical differences between true primary and nonprimary first episodes are often blurred and may be misleading—especially in pregnancy. The diagnosis should be unequivocal. This means determining that the following are true:

1. It was your first ever vaginal sore like this;

2. A herpes culture test was positive;

3. In association with a positive herpes culture, a herpes anti-body test was negative at the outset of the infection; and/or

4. Your physician feels that your symptoms were typical of primary herpes (many sores involving both sides of the genitals, lasting longer than ten days, and often associated with swollen inguinal nodes or "glands" or fever and headache).

In general, you should not have amniocentesis to find out anything about herpes. Amniocentesis can be very informative for other reasons, but amniocentesis for herpes can be misleading. Look for answers about herpes in other ways, as described above.

What can I do to prevent my baby from contracting my herpes?

Discuss herpes with your doctor early in your pregnancy. An ultrasound study early in pregnancy might be useful for determining dates. If and when the time comes for deciding whether a cesarean section is necessary, it is easiest if the doctor has all the available facts concerning when the baby is really due.

Learn the active phases of infection, monitor yourself for herpes, and report recurrences to your doctor.

If you have a symptomatic active recurrence during the last four to six weeks of pregnancy, see your doctor as soon as you can after the start of the recurrence. He or she should assess the sore and perform a culture to confirm what it is. As soon as the sore is healed, the area should be cultured again so that there is laboratory proof that the area is virus-free before you elect to have a normal vaginal birth. Guidelines from the American College of Obstetrics and Gynecology Committee recommend that every woman with a history of genital herpes have at least one negative culture before labor (with no subsequent new symptoms of active herpes) before deciding on the normal route of delivery. Yet doing weekly cultures near term without symptoms seemed to be a poor method of prevention of infection in one study in California. Studies have proven that neonatal herpes is extremely unlikely to occur, even if the mother with recurrent herpes is culture-positive during labor! The best way to prevent neonatal herpes, therefore, is an area of continuing academic controversy. I recommend that your doctor carefully examine with a strong light source the external genitals (shown in figure 6b, page 50) on your last two or three prenatal visits and once again during labor. This will let your doctor know what your genital skin normally looks like, so that he or she will be fairly confident that the appearance is normal during labor before electing to assist with a vaginal birth. A virus culture, using one moistened swab of all of the external genital areas, should be taken on at least one of the prenatal visits and repeated during labor. If a sore or symptoms of a sore are present at labor, a cesarean section is indicated. If all looks well, and the last virus culture is negative, a cesarean is not required.

Unless there is a very important reason for using one, a fetal scalp monitor should probably be avoided if you have a history of herpes.

Obtain a cesarean section if and only if you have *active* herpes or you have just had active herpes that your doctor thinks might not be healed when you go into labor. The decision about whether herpes is healed can be a tough one. Essentially we are considering the active phases (chapter 3) as active and the inactive as inactive. A culture is especially useful in keeping the time to a minimum. If the episode near the end of term is a *primary* one, it would be wise to extend the safety period because of the high risk of asymptomatic viral shedding following primary infection. I tend to use systemic acyclovir to treat primary herpes in late pregnancy and continue to use acyclovir for suppression of herpes until delivery. Because the risk of asymptomatic shedding on the cervix is very high during the few months following a first episode of genital herpes, I recommend cesarean section for most cases of true primary or nonprimary type 2 herpes infection during the third trimester.

If your herpes is active, a cesarean section is urgently needed once membranes rupture. The operation can be arranged less urgently after the onset of labor if the membranes are intact. If herpes is not active, a cesarean is not necessary.

Does a cesarean delivery always prevent transmission?

Because herpes is generally transmitted by direct contact, when a physical barrier (the bag of waters) remains between a herpes sore and a baby's skin, the risk of neonatal infection is extremely small. Thus, bypassing an active sore by delivering the baby through the abdomen (cesarean section) is an extremely effective method of prevention. Whether or not you will need a cesarean section depends on whether you are in an active phase of infection when labor begins. The statistical likelihood of needing a cesarean section will depend on how often you get recurrences. As far as we know, a high recurrence frequency rate will not detrimentally affect the risk to your baby. First episode genital infection during pregnancy, especially late pregnancy, is a different matter and is discussed elsewhere in this chapter.

Once the sac of waters is broken, the possibility of direct transmission to the baby becomes more likely. If this occurs without your knowing it (there may be small holes that heal up without symptoms), then a cesarean section may not prevent infection. The practical risk of membranes rupturing without your knowledge and causing problems is very small, however.

Confusion might arise in identifying when the bag of waters breaks; leaky fluid is usually obvious, but sudden clear fluid discharges in late pregnancy need checking out at a hospital. Once the membranes rupture—and this may be the first symptom of labor—it is only a matter of time until active herpes on the outside gets to the inside. This is because the barrier is broken and a wet path has developed. In other words, there is a fluid connection from outside to inside held nicely at body temperature, allowing the virus to find its way inside. If herpes is active on the skin when the membranes rupture, it is only a matter of time before the virus gets to the baby. Therefore, cesarean section has to be done immediately. There has been some discussion recently suggesting that it is all right to wait four hours from the time membranes rupture until the cesarean section is performed. This is not true. If herpes is considered to be active at the time the membranes rupture, a cesarean section should be performed as soon as possible.

If recurrent herpes is active and membranes have not been ruptured for a prolonged period of time, cesarean section is often the best way of helping the body in the job it is already performing of efficiently and effectively preventing herpes transmission to the newborn. Arguments are being made by health economists and statisticians and even some clinical experts, however, that would suggest holding back with cesarean section except in cases of true primary or nonprimary type 2 genital infection. For now, I prefer to stick with the long-practiced approach of recommending cesarean section if there is evidence of an active episode of recurrent herpes. Chances are, though, that the newborn baby will be healthy regardless of which path the woman with recurrent herpes and her doctor choose. First episodes of genital herpes during late pregnancy are a different matter and need specialized care.

Why don't all pregnant women with genital herpes have cesarean sections?

Some pregnant women with herpes feel that cesarean is the way to go regardless of the situation. Often this stems from the burden of guilt that the woman feels would arise from an infection in the baby. This is a very noble thought indeed, but it is often based on a lack of understanding of the facts. Here are the facts:

1. Genital herpes is a common problem, while neonatal herpes is an uncommon one.

2. A cesarean section may be needed if herpes is active during labor. Even in those cases of recurrent herpes where we have traditionally considered cesarean section necessary, however, medical experts and epidemiologists are beginning to question this approach. While it still remains the current standard of medical practice to recommend cesarean section during an active genital recurrence, there is little proof that this approach significantly improves the natural protection conferred by the woman's own immunity and the limited lesion area exposure found during a mild recurrence. If we are beginning to question the validity of cesarean section during an active episode, it makes even less sense to opt for cesarean section when herpes is inactive. With the exception of the post-first episode, if episodes of recurrent genital herpes are not active during labor, cesarean section offers no advantages over normal vaginal birth.

3. Despite its overall good safety record, the risk of cesarean section to the mother is much higher than that of vaginal birth.

After all, cesarean birth is a form of surgery. It means a longer hospital stay and a higher risk of postpartum (after birth) complications to the mother, such as fever and infection. The risk of cesarean section is low, but the risks of surgery clearly outweigh any potential benefits when herpes is not active at the time of labor.

4. Even cesarean section won't necessarily prevent neonatal herpes, which can come from other sources than the mother's genital herpes—for example, transmission of herpes from Aunt Sadie's fever blister. It is much better to think out the problem and use care in avoiding transmission. A prevention panacea may just obscure the issues.

If acyclovir is probably safe during pregnancy, why can't I take it to prevent the need for cesarean section?

This technique is under study, and initial data suggest that this may be a very effective approach. (Antiviral treatment in general is further discussed in chapter 11.) The official stand is that treatment is not advised until further studies show that this approach is safe and effective. To date, the studies performed have not been large enough to draw complete conclusions. As discussed earlier in this chapter, oral acyclovir is probably safe in pregnancy. Since the indication for cesarean section is the appearance of a clinical recurrence of herpes during labor, and since acyclovir suppression has been shown to reduce the rates of clinical recurrence dramatically, it follows that acyclovir suppression would markedly reduce the number of cesarean sections performed for herpes recurrences. If no harm came to the mother or baby, then this cost-effective use of medication would be of great benefit, since it would limit the duration of hospitalization and complications from the cesarean sections done for herpes. It will be virtually impossible to prove that this suppressive approach is effective at reducing the rate of neonatal herpes, since in most cases mothers with first episode genital herpes infection are not undergoing any drug intervention or serial assessment. There just aren't enough cases to show that any treatment would prevent disease in the baby.

There are several possible negative aspects to acyclovir treatment during late pregnancy:

1. This treatment has not been proven safe in pregnancy. It is possible that some hidden side effects of treatment in pregnancy will emerge later. There are theoretical concerns that kidney damage or reduced white blood cell counts in the newborn might occur.

2. There is no evidence to favor the idea that taking acyclovir might protect the baby from getting herpes. It would be used, instead, to improve the likelihood of the pregnant woman having a vaginal delivery. Thus, there is no guarantee that the use of acyclovir (or any other drug) will prevent newborns from getting herpes.

3. Neonatal herpes occurred in one baby in a study where acyclovir suppression was used for this purpose.

4. It is possible that suppression with acyclovir could mask a recurrence without fully preventing viral shedding. It is thus theoretically possible that acyclovir treatment might actually increase the chance of missing an active episode and exposing the baby to active virus.

Despite these possible negatives, there are a lot of potential positives that warrant consideration of this approach. Probably the strongest positive reason suggesting that acyclovir suppression may be sensible in late pregnancy is its positive effect on reducing asymptomatic viral shedding. But until definitive data prove the correct approach, I believe that the potential benefit could be very good, assuming that definitive clinical trials support some of the preliminary information suggesting that this approach may reduce the cesarean section rate. Unfortunately, the safety of this treatment is unproven. Therefore, if a pregnant woman wishes, and if she understands that this is not a proven area, and especially if she has high recurrence frequency rates that are very likely to require her to have a cesarean section, I would proceed carefully, using 1,000 to 1,200 mg per day in three to six doses. I would still recommend cesarean section for an active episode, and I would still like to see the mother cultured during labor and the baby cultured after birth for herpes to be sure nothing was missed. Whenever a drug is used outside of the list of possible indications from the FDA (or its equivalent in your country) it becomes an area of hot controversy. On the one hand, physicians and patients need to be able to proceed on the basis of best clinical judgment in areas where treatment is likely to work. On the other hand, we do not know with certainty that the treatment as described in this chapter is effective. Sometimes expensive, ineffective, or even harmful treatments get entrenched without proof into common clinical practice. For now, there is the clear possibility that treatment could turn out to be worse than no treatment. On the other hand, to miss the chance at having a normal vaginal birth while waiting for the data to become available is also a potential unnecessary loss. Discuss the issues with your doctor. Do not take it upon yourself, under any circumstances, to use acyclovir during pregnancy or otherwise, without the prescription of your doctor for this express purpose. Using this drug, like any other drug, requires care and correct understanding of what to expect in light of a full understanding of your own health. Couples and friends sometimes share drugs without the input of their doctor. This is never recommended and is especially unwise during pregnancy.

Is there treatment for an affected baby?

Yes. (Antiviral treatment in general is discussed in chapter 11.) We now have very effective means of killing the virus while it is active. Our problems, in general, in devising new ways to kill herpes are twofold. First, therapy cannot undo damage already done to vital structures, although it can probably stop progression of damage from the infection. Second, it does not alter latent infection (see chapter 1), and therefore virus infection may recur. Suspected neonatal herpes should be quickly and aggressively diagnosed. If a newborn baby becomes ill and the mother has a history of herpes, she should make sure that the pediatrician knows of her history. If the father or any other sexual partner has herpes, that fact is also important, since the mother could then have herpes without knowing it. Remember, too, that neonatal herpes can occur even where both parents have never knowingly had a herpes sore of any kind. Make sure someone explains to you how the possibilities of herpes (and other problems) are being investigated. If herpes is not a consideration to the physician, is that because there is a good reason not to consider it? It is certainly possible to have good medical reasons not to consider the diagnosis of herpes in a newborn, but you should suggest looking for herpes just to make sure that your doctor has thought of the possibility. If your doctor does not consider herpes a possibility, he or she should explain why not.

Adenine arabinoside (ara-A, Vira-A) and acyclovir (Zovirax) are both very useful agents for treating neonatal herpes. Both are effective agents at reducing the disease, regardless of the type of disease at the outset of treatment. Most physicians choose to use acyclovir because it has far fewer side effects and is easier to administer. Neither agent can reverse tissue damage that has already occurred. Physicians' ability to diagnose neonatal herpes more quickly and at much milder stages than in years past is improving the prognosis for newborns quite dramatically. Still, the diagnosis is all too often made after some irreversible harm has already come to the newborn baby. New data also suggest that after a successful initial treatment period with intravenous acyclovir, continuous dosing with oral acyclovir syrup is sometimes recommended after proven neonatal herpes infection, depending on the type and severity of the baby's illness. We need to focus on prevention, but prevention is needed most where it is applied the least—i.e., where the mother does *not* think she has genital herpes.

Occasionally a baby is treated with acyclovir when there is no illness whatsoever, if after a normal vaginal delivery or prolonged membrane rupture it is discovered that the baby has already been exposed. Such a chance exposure to a sore could occur if a sore is noticed only after delivery or in the unlikely event of asymptomatic virus shedding. Although no scientific studies have been performed to support the use of acyclovir in this setting, and many experts in this field prefer not to use the drug in this setting, acyclovir is often used in the newborn if the mother's infection was her first. In a recent report, 12 (46 percent) of 26 newborns who were treated early in infancy and then kept on acyclovir for months after, experienced a reduction in their white blood cell counts. Although this has not been shown to be a clinical problem for the infants, it does point out that the use of any drug, especially in early infancy or childhood, needs to be undertaken only with the careful advice, prescription, and follow-up of a physician. This and other medical issues need to be considered in discussion with your baby's physician. In the future, we may be able to further protect the infant with vaccines for the mother and/or the infant as well as more potent medicines. Even without these safeguards, however, the vast majority of newborn babies of women with recurrent genital herpes do not need any more protection than nature provides.

If I have active herpes during labor, can I have epidural anesthesia?

Yes, unless your herpes is a true primary. In that situation, there is a slight risk to the mother of herpes meningitis (see chapter 3), which *might* cause complications from the epidural. In that very unusual case, the anesthetist may wish to opt for a general anesthetic during the cesarean section. Because of this *theoretical risk*, some anesthetists have opted for general anesthetic even during recurrent episodes of genital herpes. Recurrent herpes has never been associated in any way with any proven risk increase after epidural anesthesia. Drs. Ramanathan, Sheth, and Turndorf first published their findings about this in the journal *Anesthesiology* in 1986. They studied 56 women in labor with genital herpes infection, 33 of whom had epidural anesthesia. No complications related to the anesthetic developed in either group. In addition, Drs. Crosby, Halpern, and Rolbin reported their findings in 1989 in the *Canadian Journal of Anaesthesia.* To quote their review of six years' experience in the use of epidural anesthesia at Toronto's Women's College Hospital, "No patient suffered an adverse outcome related to either the anaesthetic or the virus. The theoretical risks of regional anaesthesia in the parturient [woman giving birth] with active herpes genitalis are reviewed. We conclude from available data that the risk of an adverse outcome is small and does not contraindicate the use of epidural anaesthesia in patients with recurrent infection." Active recurrent or inactive recurrent genital herpes does not contraindicate epidural anesthesia.

What are my baby's chances of getting herpes?

Neonatal herpes is very unlikely to occur in an infant born to a woman who has genital herpes and knows she has it. By contrast, if the woman does not know she has genital herpes, and especially if the infection occurs for the first time during labor, the baby is at much greater risk. A woman with recurrent infection is unlikely to transmit infection for the following reasons:

1. Any recurrence of herpes is likely to have virus present on the involved area of skin for only a short time. In a closely monitored study in Vancouver, we found that without any special treatment, 50 percent of women with recurrent herpes stopped shedding virus entirely within 56 hours after onset of symptoms. In other words, as soon as virus appears on the skin, nature is already effectively getting rid of it.

2. The mother's immunity to herpes is transferred, in part, to the newborn, offering protection from minor exposure. Babies born to mothers with recurrent herpes have a lot of antibody to herpes. The mother is likely to have high levels of anti-herpes antibody that will be passed on to the baby and the amniotic fluid surrounding the baby, thereby neutralizing the virus in most cases before it has a chance to get into the epithelial cells of the newborn infant.

3. The mother's herpes sore is usually localized, external, and far away from the birth canal, and the cervix is usually free of infection.

4. The mother's recurrent herpes does not make her systemically ill, so the baby is not subject to health problems in the mother.

5. The amount of virus in a recurrent sore is quite small compared with the amount present in primary infection and so is less likely to get to the newborn and cause infection.

6. During primary infection, sores may continue to have active virus present for days or even weeks. Virus in a recurrent sore, however, is present for only a short period of time.

7. The mother has a greater than 95 percent chance of knowing on the basis of her symptoms whether she is culture-positive and potentially exposing the baby. If symptoms of an active phase of infection are present, she will be able to have a cesarean section.

8. Most babies who are exposed to the virus do not actually acquire infection, for the reasons listed above. Of those who do, the vast majority do not develop disease as a result.

9. If exposure to virus has occurred, the physician may choose to treat the baby with a very effective antiviral agent, acyclovir (oral or intravenous). Because the chances of the baby getting sick are so low, even after an episode of obvious exposure to virus, many physicians choose not to use acyclovir. This is an area of academic controversy. I favor treatment before disease develops, in an attempt to prevent this from happening, although I recognize that the clinical trials that have been performed to examine this question are inadequate from the scientific point of view to prove safety and benefit. It may be a very long time before enough patients can be studied to absolutely prove that this approach is beneficial. To me, it just makes clinical sense.

Physicians must make an educated guess that a pregnant woman with recurrent genital herpes will give birth to a baby with a herpes infection, because accurate statistics do not exist. The risk is probably less than one in several thousands that this will happen to any individual with recurrent genital herpes so long as the usual guidelines are followed. The risk of herpes is thus no greater than the risk of a variety of other neonatal diseases. Herpes should not prevent you from having children should you elect to do so.

Crystal ball? In the future, we will probably be suppressing herpes shedding late in pregnancy with safe and effective medications that block the transmission of virus. Screening for herpes will be universal, not limited to women who know they have herpes. Women who are at risk of getting herpes during pregnancy will be protected by vaccine taken before conception or possibly during pregnancy. Where it is not known if the woman is at risk, and thus the neonate may be at risk, the baby will be vaccinated to prevent infection at birth.

7
Herpes
and Cancer

Who cares about your questions, you still won't be going
back home. You may as well give back your glasses.
And your pajamas.

—ALEKSANDR SOLZHENITSYN
Cancer Ward

Are herpes and cancer related?

Although some of the human herpes viruses do cause cancer, there is no proof that herpes simplex does. A scientific argument about the causes of cervical cancer still exists, however. Let us review the evidence. First of all, did you know that sex causes cancer? This is not even controversial. Sex is associated with cancers that result from the transmission of human immunodeficiency virus (HIV). People with HIV who develop AIDS quite frequently develop cancers as a result of their immunodeficiency. These cancers include Kaposi's sarcoma (caused by human herpes virus type 8), lymphoma, and certain squamous cell cancers. In some cases, the cause of an AIDS-related tumor is infection, in that the immunodeficiency has reduced the person's ability to fight the infection normally in order to prevent the cancer.

Even without the transmission of HIV, however, sex is associated with cancer of the cervix and of the vulva. Cancer of the cervix is a common tumor in prostitutes, rare in Catholic nuns. It occurs more often in women who begin having first sexual contact early and who have more sexual partners. It is not surprising, then, to find that one sexually transmitted agent, namely herpes simplex, is more common in women with cervical cancer than in those without. About twenty-five years ago, studies began to show over and over again a *seroepidemiologic* association between the two diseases. This means that a blood, or serum ("sero-"), test for antibodies to herpes simplex type 2 is positive more often in groups ("-epidemiologic") of women *with* cancer than in groups without. By themselves, however, these studies tell us little. Sex causes cervical cancer. Furthermore, sex predisposes an individual to getting genital herpes. So it is no surprise to find that both herpes and cancer of the cervix have been found to be more common in women who have more sex-related risk factors. It would have been more surprising not to find this.

The *human papillomavirus* (HPV), known to cause venereal warts, has also been called an *oncogenic* (cancer-causing) virus. Evidence now overwhelmingly points to this virus as the true cervical cancer virus. Certain subtypes are very closely related to cancer development.

As we get better and better at detecting and probing for causes, invasive cancer of the cervix is becoming less and less common. Early Pap smear changes are often treated so quickly that cancer is never allowed to develop.

The Pap smear is an important health tool for any woman who has been sexually active. Early detection means that cervical cancer is unlikely to develop, and an abnormality is very easy to detect before it becomes cancerous. If cancer does develop, it starts out very slowly, allowing lots of time to take successful curative action during the early stages. The Pap smear is used for detection—use it regularly.

Cancer of the vulva, the woman's external genitals, is also a slow-growing cancer. It is much less common than cancer of the cervix. It is now also known to be caused by human papillomavirus. The symptoms are commonly external itching, pain, or the observance of a growth. Its most common locations—on the external genitals—parallel those of genital herpes. Although itching of the vaginal area is seldom related to cancer, persistent vaginal itching should be explored for possible causes. See your physician if you are concerned.

If I have herpes, is it on the cervix? Inside the vagina?

During primary genital herpes, nine out of ten women with herpes on the labia also have herpes on the cervix. Sometimes this may cause *cervicitis*, or inflammation of the cervix with an associated vaginal discharge. Sores can develop on the cervix as well. Herpes is probably a cause of nonspecific cervicitis more often than is realized. Cervicitis and discharge are common during primary herpes, even in the absence of external sores—sometimes because external sores develop a bit later in the course of infection and sometimes because external sores never develop during primary herpes.

During recurrences of genital herpes, herpes on the cervix is uncommon. A carefully performed study has shown that herpes can be recovered from the cervix in only 4 percent of recurrent cases. In fact, it may be that many of these were not really on the cervix but appeared to be there because of the "wet path" that exists between cervix and sore. It is impossible to examine the cervix without first touching the vulva and entrance to the vagina—typical external areas of recurrent infection. Genital herpes is an external infection for the most part. In women, it occurs mainly on the vaginal lips, the perianal area, the perineum (between anus and vagina) and the pubic region. The cervix is an uncommon site of infection during recurrences.

What are my chances of getting cervical cancer?

There are different degrees of cervical cancer, according to epidemiologists who look at the problem and according to the women affected by this disease. Cancer detected on a Pap smear before any damage whatsoever is done to the person occurs in about 1 in 1,000 women over the age of twenty. Depending on the study, the risk increases to 2 to 8 per 1,000 women with genital herpes. Other factors, such as smoking cigarettes may also increase the risk of developing cancer of the cervix. Clinically significant cervical cancer (one that has gone far enough that it might do harm to the person if not dealt with immediately) occurs with much less frequency (closer to 7 or 8 of 100,000 women over the age of twenty). The risk of this type of cancer occurring in people with genital herpes increases to approximately 15 to 100 cases per 100,000 women over the age of twenty probably because, overall, people with herpes are statistically more likely to also have infection with human papillomavirus. The average age of occurrence is the late forties, although cervical cancer can be seen as early as the teens or as late as the eighties. The responsible virus is not herpes. But people who have herpes also have human papillomavirus more than other people do.

What should I do to prevent cervical cancer from becoming a problem?

A *Pap smear* is a simple procedure and should be part of your annual gynecological examination. It is quick and simple to do correctly. The best time to have it done is just before or at ovulation, when estrogen hormone levels are high and the cells are flatter and easier to interpret under the microscope. The test can also be done at any other time if ovulation is an inconvenient time to make the visit to the physician. First, a plastic or metal speculum is inserted into the vagina, as pictured in figure 10. This allows the examiner to see the cervix by gently pushing the walls of the vagina aside. Any vaginal discharge and cervical mucus coating the cervix are then swabbed away using a cotton swab. A wooden scraper shaped like a stretched Popsicle stick is used to scrape cells from the surface of the cervix onto a slide, which is then sent to the laboratory.

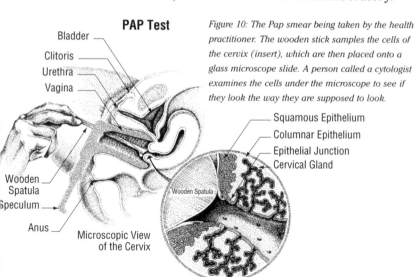

PAP Test

Bladder
Clitoris
Urethra
Vagina

Squamous Epithelium
Columnar Epithelium
Epithelial Junction
Cervical Gland

Wooden Spatula

Wooden Spatula
Speculum

Anus

Microscopic View of the Cervix

Figure 10: The Pap smear being taken by the health practitioner. The wooden stick samples the cells of the cervix (insert), which are then placed onto a glass microscope slide. A person called a cytologist examines the cells under the microscope to see if they look the way they are supposed to look.

The Pap smear detects any unusual cells from the cervix. If cells are cancerous, it will detect them. If cells are just upset from infection, it will detect them also. All of these cells will be called abnormal. Since cancer of the cervix is very slow to grow, a yearly Pap smear is an adequate test. Some physicians feel that Pap smears are needed less frequently. As long as they stay normal—Class 1— one per year is plenty. If your Pap smear is abnormal in any way, more frequent smears may be appropriate. If you have had several normal Pap smears on a yearly basis and you are not changing sexual partners and your sexual partner is not changing sexual partners, then it may be appropriate to have Pap smears performed less often. Discuss these issues with your physician.

Whether you have herpes or not, the yearly Pap smear *is* a good idea however. Rest assured that if you follow this regimen, any detected cancer of the cervix is likely to be curable. I recommend putting this cancer issue out of your mind except for one big red mark on each new calendar—the day for your yearly Pap test.

My Pap smear is abnormal. What does that mean?

The Pap smear is a method of examining the cells that line the cervix. Anything that changes those cells will change your Pap smear. During primary herpes, a Pap smear is abnormal from infection but changes back to normal after the primary episode has cleared; this abnormal smear is of no concern. Other infections— such as *trichomoniasis*, *bacterial vaginosis*, and *gonorrhea*—may also change the Pap smear. In each case, if the Pap has become abnormal as a symptom of infection, treatment of the infection will cause the Pap to revert to normal eventually. A Pap will also be abnormal if cancer of the cervix has developed. It is obviously important to find out if your abnormal Pap is from infection or cancer. How is this done?

Pap abnormalities are classified. The classifications vary from city to city, state to state, province to province, and country to country. There are scores ranging from normal to obvious invasive cancer, with many gray areas in between. If the score is abnormal, there are several things to do. If the most severely abnormal condition is detected, indicating invasive cancer, a *colposcopy* is generally performed. If a less severely abnormal condition is discovered, your best bet is first to make sure that all possible infections have been ruled out. Your doctor will do (or may already have done) a culture test for Chlamydia, gonorrhea, and Candida. A microscopic examination for *Trichomonas vaginalis* and an assessment for bacterial vaginosis are also performed. If your abnormal Pap was taken during or shortly after your primary herpes, you may also want to repeat the test to see if the situation has improved on its own. If another infection is present, have the Pap test done again two or three months later to see if it has returned to normal.

Let's say you still have an abnormal test. If an infection was present, you've had it treated. You've waited several months. If the score shows only a mild abnormality, you will likely be advised to wait and see and to have another test in a few months. Probably, this abnormal score will eventually vanish. If your score shows consistently abnormal cells, you may be sent for a colposcopy test. This is an examination of the cervix much like the Pap smear. The speculum exam is repeated, as for the Pap smear. Then the physician inserts a microscope-like instrument through the speculum to take a very close look at the surface of the cervix. Biopsies are taken for further laboratory examination. A biopsy of the cervix may feel like a pinch or may not be felt at all. The procedure is very, very safe. A small amount of bleeding is to be expected. The laboratory examines the biopsies and offers an opinion. If invasive or microinvasive cancer is present on a biopsy, the therapy is removal of the cancer. Surgery may be required. The most common surgery is the *cone biopsy*, in which only the inner core of the cervix is removed through the vagina. Generally, a cone biopsy does not prevent either sexual intercourse or normal birth.

The different possible therapies to be chosen at this point are beyond the scope of this book. If your biopsy is in a less severe category, arguments exist about what therapy you should have. You may be advised in one center to have a cone biopsy for severe dysplasia (abnormal tissue growth), and in another center to wait, see, and repeat for *carcinoma in situ*. Why all the conflicting advice? Most cervices in this gray area will not progress to invasive cancer, if left alone. Many will revert to a normal condition with no intervention. However, many physicians argue that most is not good enough.

The safest (and most invasive) thing to do with cervical tissue diagnosed as being in a gray area is to remove it from the cervix. Have you ever been asked if you see the proverbial glass of water as half full or half empty? The right course of action is not cast in stone: if the situation should arise, discuss it at length with your doctor and read a lot more on the topic. Keep in mind that if you have an abnormal result from a routine Pap smear, you have found the problem early and can get treatment that is effective and safe!

8

The Psychology of Herpes

*[I]t is hardly possible to take up one's residence in the
kingdom of the ill unprejudiced by the lurid metaphors
with which it has been landscaped.*

—SUSAN SONTAG
Illness as Metaphor

What are some of the common emotional reactions to herpes?

How does herpes affect your life? Is it a minor health issue you face
directly or a major disturbance in your day-to-day life? Many people who have herpes become very distressed by the impact of
transmission, asymptomatic shedding, partner discussions and
the irritations of recurrences in their lives. I often ask people "If
you were to rank the top ten things of importance in your life in
order of importance, would herpes be on the list?" Many of my
patients answer yes and some even rank herpes number one. If
herpes is on your list, I hope that your goal will be to reduce its
rank or even get it off the list. It is important to ask how a minor
skin ailment that affects a quarter of the population and rarely
affects a person's overall health manages to gain such importance
to so many people. If herpes does rank high on your list, perhaps
some ideas from this chapter will help to knock it down a few pegs.

Herpes causes a spectrum of physical distress that ranges from
asymptomatic (no symptoms) to very severe. The physical symptoms of herpes are not the same for everyone. Similarly, the emotional impact of herpes cannot be typified, categorized, or
compartmentalized. The emotional effect depends to some extent

on how severely herpes affects you physically. A painful and prolonged primary infection might result in a severe reaction of shock and anger. Any emotional reaction will also depend on how you were informed of the diagnosis. Was the person knowledgeable? Judgmental? Informative? What were your preconceived ideas about herpes? Did you learn about herpes before you became infected, and were you prepared for the possibility, or did you think it could never happen to you? Is your background a religious one? Did you believe that herpes was a punishment visited on those who have it? Have you known other people with herpes? What were their emotional and physical reactions to herpes? What have their experiences been with this infection? Can you accept the inevitable, generally? Do you know how you got herpes? Do you feel guilt or shame about the circumstances under which you became infected? Do you feel hurt by the person who transmitted herpes to you? Has herpes disrupted your lifestyle? By how much? Are you afraid of getting involved because you will have to tell your partner? Do you feel that you have been victimized?

Some of the more common reactions to herpes are described below. Some are only temporary; others have lasting impact. You should not necessarily expect to experience any of these reactions. Whether or not you do, you are not alone with your feelings.

On first learning about herpes, you may have a feeling of shock. There may be a sudden change in the image you have of your own body, or you may have a sense of loss. Some people react with panic when they hear the word "herpes," which they associate with other words such as "contagious" and "incurable." You might feel this during a severe primary infection, when you are ill and terribly uncomfortable. You may have been told that you have herpes but have been informed of little else. You may have heard that herpes is painful or incurable, and may imagine (incorrectly) either that this primary herpes will recur with the same intensity or that it will go on forever.

Shock may also be your response if the diagnosis has been unexpected. You may have gone to the doctor because of something like a recurring yeast infection, hemorrhoids, or a spider bite, only to be told you have genital herpes. You may feel trapped inside a defective body over which you have lost control. Regaining emo tional and physical control requires regrouping your thoughts. Adjusting to having herpes cannot be instantaneous. It comes through experience, study, and observation. People with herpes should strive toward normalization, a process that requires time in which to gain perspective. Normalization comes through an active process of learning the facts about herpes and, just as important, passing through the stage of self-pity toward an ability to work with those facts.

At first, the diagnosis of herpes may be frightening. Everyone knows that herpes is common, but some people choose to believe that the lack of current press attention means that herpes is not a current problem. Nobody expects to get herpes—just as venereal disease in general is thought of as something that *other* people get. You may have feared getting herpes and now you may fear having it. Once you understand it, though, you can see that the physical symptoms do not threaten your life, your sanity, or your health. You can certainly be sexually healthy, physically healthy, and mentally healthy, *and have genital herpes.*

Until the facts are clear, fear may well be your dominant emotional reaction to your herpes. It may be difficult to relate to others while you are afraid. You may want to seek out unrealistic cures rather than to face the issues directly. This may arise in part from the difficulty of finding material to read that does not scare you even more. Alternatively, you may have come across material that reassures you beyond what is believable. You may not yet have had a health practitioner explain the details of herpes to you. Herpes is a well-characterized, recurrent viral infection that you can fully understand. Being in possession of all the facts will help put things into perspective.

You may feel shame about having a "social disease." This shame may be amplified by the jokes of your friends or by the expressions of their own fears. A feeling may predominate that there is something shameful to hide. In fact, you may not wish to discuss herpes with some people. Herpes is like any other secret. Because its origin is in sexual contact, you may feel strongly about keeping herpes a secret—private, discreet. This may reflect how you feel about the sexual encounter that you feel resulted in herpes.

However, any anxiety you feel because you are keeping the secret should be distinguished in your mind from any feeling of shame for having acquired herpes. Whom you tell is up to you. Some people feel the need to talk about herpes to casual friends. This may make things feel more acceptable to you or may give you allies who condone the situation. But do not rely on other people to give you peace of mind. Confession does not solve the problem. Under some circumstances, confession of some kind may be appropriate or even necessary. For instance, you may need to clear the air and discuss a love affair, because having herpes has made it difficult *not* to discuss it. A religious person may feel the need for absolution. One confesses the deed, however, not the virus.

It is critical to separate the deed from the virus. Good deeds or bad, right deeds or wrong, happy deeds or sad—these definitions are left to the philosopher and the theologian. The moral choices are left to the individual. Viruses are another matter. Viruses are in the realm of the virologist, the physician, and the epidemiologist. Viruses do not make moral choices. We regard them as bad because they cause sores and are parasitic. Viruses do not choose on whom they land on the basis of moral principles. For instance, before the advent of polio vaccine twenty-five years ago, the polio virus paralyzed countless thousands of children each year. There was nothing moral or immoral about this phenomenon; it was simply the result of the nature of the virus and the susceptibility of children. Similarly, herpes may be passed by contact from the mouth of a mother to the eye of her child because of the most innocent and morally correct act—a loving kiss. Herpes sores on the genitals of an adult are no more issues of morality than are herpes sores on the mouth of a child. Shame has nothing to do with the biological facts of this virus. If you are being honest and clear about your herpes with your partner, you owe no one an apology.

Alternatively, a feeling of guilt may result from the nature of the sexual involvement. You may also feel guilty because of your potential to transmit herpes—a problem minimized by education, awareness, and open and frank discussions with sexual partners. Occasionally, people with herpes find themselves in the position of soothing the guilt of the partner who transmitted the infection. People who get herpes from a partner may also feel guilty for getting the infection—especially when the partner who transmitted herpes is asymptomatic. Now that the Western blot test is available, the facts can often help to figure out the situation.

Anger is a common reaction to herpes. Initial feelings of shock or subsequent feelings of guilt may give way to anger. Anger is a normal response to a loss. Herpes has invaded your domain. Even though you know that active phases follow a cycle, you have to accept the fact that it is not possible to eradicate the virus itself and that there are no complete guarantees about transmission. A feeling of frustration is understandable.

Anger may also be directed at the person who transmitted the infection to you; you may feel tainted, betrayed, compromised, or perhaps even abandoned. The overwhelming majority of people who transmit herpes fall into one of these categories:

1. They did not know what the sores (or cuts, or slits, or pimples, or whatever) were.

2. They have never had any symptoms suggestive of herpes.

3. They knew about the presence of herpes but were mistaken about the active phases of infection.

4. They had shown the sores to a health care practitioner who said the sores were nothing to worry about.

5. They were tested for herpes and the virus culture was negative, and they did not understand what this meant.

6. They understood the active phases of infection, were careful, and still transmitted the infection because of asymptomatic shedding.

None of the six categories describes evil people with "malice aforethought." Though conscientious and careful, a person with herpes may have been told that herpes was "just a virus infection" or "just a cold sore of the genitals." They may not have realized the need to avoid transmission or known the best methods of doing so. In fact, most partners of people who have just contracted primary genital herpes deny any history of herpes, not because they are liars, but because symptoms have never suggested that herpes is present. Many people with herpes are misinformed. The person who knew about his or her herpes infection and failed to tell may not have had enough courage or enough medical information to properly explain the problem. Perhaps he or she was inarticulate, shy, or was afraid to tamper with the relationship. Perhaps telling a previous partner resulted in a traumatic breakup. In many cases, people are most afraid to tell the partners they most care about. The person with herpes is in a confusing position with a tough responsibility. If you find yourself temporarily despising the person who gave you herpes, vent your anger in other ways. If you are sure who gave you herpes, tell the person, but try not to hurt him or her. It may be a difficult time for him or her also. Often anger directed at the person who you think gave you herpes results from a misunderstanding of how transmission occurs. Later you might find yourself turning your anger inward for being "foolish" enough to catch herpes. This is a more destructive form of anger. If you are angry at a friend, the friend can walk away, but it is more difficult to walk away from yourself. Try to place your anger correctly in the lap of the virus. In other words, remember the distinction between virus and deed. Herpes is a reality for all people who have sexual contact.

Your anger may also be directed at the health professional who informs you of the diagnosis. He or she is also the one who fails to offer you a cure, and you may see this as the worst sin of all. Every health care professional must be prepared for this. If the physician's answers to patients' questions are thoughtful and informed, anger and frustration will be minimized. If the physician makes the mistake of sitting in judgment or of providing inadequate information, anger directed against the physician can be expected.

Depression is a common emotional reaction to herpes. Many people are understandably depressed by having the infection. Anyone would rather not have herpes. Depression may result from the frustration of having an "incurable" disease. A sense of hopelessness arises in some people with each active recurrence. Very frequent recurrences may cause a repeating sequence of anger and depression while the person is trying to cope with the actual physical distress of the recurrences. It is normal to feel depressed over having herpes. You now have an obligation to discuss herpes with sexual partners, to become aware of your recurrence patterns and avoid sore contact during active phases, and to monitor child-birth. This means some loss of spontaneity and freedom. Depression may also result from a loss of self-esteem—a feeling that you will never be perfect or that you have not lived up to your expectations. The self-esteem tied up in our sexuality can be threatened by the fear of transmitting herpes or by concern over temporary skin discoloration. Sexual acts leave the participants vulnerable. When herpes complicates this vulnerability, there may be a tendency to feel wronged. Isolation may follow in order to protect a person from further losses. Isolation carried to an extreme, however, can result in a feeling of being a sexual leper—a feeling that one is alone and *should* be alone.

It is common for people with herpes to feel victimized. Indeed, some people who feel victimized are suing their source partners. In situations such as rape or intentional herpes transmission, one person clearly is victimized. Although feeling victimized is under-standable, it can also be self-destructive, and it will not help you to get your life back together. Getting control of your life means learn-ing to step out of the suit of armor of the victim and taking over the driver's seat of your life once again—regardless of whether you were truly victimized by herpes.

In some people, depression becomes overwhelming, and a healthy degree of sadness changes to a feeling of hopelessness. At this point, depression becomes a problem on its own, in addition to herpes. It may be difficult to tell where predictable feelings about an upsetting thing like herpes end and clinical depression begins. Clinical depression is an unusual reaction to herpes, how-ever. If it does occur, it may make you feel as if life's efforts are futile. Most (but not all) people who are clinically depressed feel "blue" or low, so low that it becomes increasingly difficult to enjoy life and to have good times. Their appetite may decrease or increase, they may lose or gain weight, and they may feel a loss of their normal body energy and vitality. Sleep patterns may be inter-rupted by difficulty in falling asleep (tossing and turning) or by awakening in the middle of the night and not being able to get back to sleep. Depression may also lead to loss of the usual drive at work. Sexual desire may disappear. It may become difficult to concentrate. There may be thoughts of suicide or even a plan for how to commit suicide. Other manifestations of clinical depression are aches and pains that have no physical cause and phobias—fear of heights or fear of closed spaces, for example. If symptoms of depression take on importance of their own in your life, apart from herpes—especially if several of these symptoms occur together—then you owe it to yourself to treat the depression seriously. Clinical depression can happen to anyone, with herpes or not, and should not go unchecked. If you think you might be clinically depressed, seek help—it is treatable.

Can emotions trigger a recurrence?

Triggers for herpes are discussed in chapter 3. The acknowledged triggers are all different types of stressors (anything, whether good or bad, that causes stress). Stressors include such things as menstrual periods, fever, immunosuppression from chemotherapy treatments, surgery, and even direct sunlight to the affected area. Most people feel that one stressor or another is responsible for triggering *some* recurrences. However, the overwhelming majority of herpes recurrences in any one individual happen for no apparent reason. They occur without relation to stressors and without changes in immunity. Recurrences just happen. People who are undergoing a high degree of emotional stress may have more recurrences than those who are not. However, numerous factors that are difficult to categorize or control may interact at any moment to trigger a recurrence.

There is little scientific evidence to support the idea that controlling emotional stressors diminishes herpes recurrences—or decreases the chance of having a heart attack or of getting an ulcer, for that matter. Every effort should be made, however, to take control of the stressors in your life, not because you can count on a reduction in herpes recurrences but because life is, by its nature, a series of stressful events of which herpes infection is one. Newspapers and magazines tend to make stress control and coping with herpes seem synonymous. This is not based on fact but rather on the hope that new stress control methods will help to diminish recurrences of herpes. People with herpes often believe, based on personal experience, that stress is a trigger. Some people say that having to tell your partner you have herpes is enough stress to trigger an outbreak. I do not wish to counter the emotional stress-trigger theory, but I would advise you to avoid feeling a sense of failure or guilt each time herpes recurs. Scientists are currently studying this area carefully, because the close relationship between latent herpes and the nervous system may have much to teach us. For now, there is no direct cause-and-effect relation between emotional stress and herpes episodes. Scientists who have studied stress with the timing of recurrent herpes episodes have not been able to make a good correlation. Furthermore, herpes is a very strong stressor in its own right. Stress control and coping methods are useful means of living with herpes. If you find that certain types of stress controls also become useful for you in keeping your recurrence rate low, then you are among the lucky.

What can I do to cope?

Use these suggestions or replace them with reasonable alternatives of your own:

1. Go to a clinic or your own doctor for diagnosis (see chapter 4). Your distress will be at least partially relieved by *knowing*. If you know for sure that you have herpes, you can deal with it logically and straightforwardly. Since lesions come and go, and since the active phases of infection are the best time for diagnosis, go to your health care provider when the lesions are just beginning. If you do not have lesions at present, go anyway to make plans for a visit during active lesions so you know when to get diagnosed by culture during the early active phase of infection or so that you can discuss alternatives to viral culture, such as the Western blot serologic test.

2. You are not alone with your herpes, and you are not alone with your feelings. Your emotional response, whether it is shock, anger, loneliness, or even despair, is something others have also experienced in this situation. People recover from this. Things will get better, especially if you are motivated to make sure that they do.

3. Face your fears directly. Expect that some aspects of herpes will bother you more than others, and learn more about those aspects. You will get through this.

4. Where appropriate, get treatment with safe and effective medications now available for herpes (see chapter 11 on treatment for more details):

   –If you have a first episode, your doctor should start treatment with one of the oral antiviral medications as soon as possible (see chapter 11). Topical treatments, herbal treatments, and other alternative therapies should not replace the correct use of oral antiviral treatment during a first episode.

   –If you are having frequent recurrent episodes, you may wish to consider taking one of the oral antiviral medications on a chronic basis to reduce the frequency of episodes.

   –If you are having infrequent but bothersome recurrent episodes, you may wish to consider taking one of the new oral antiviral medicines that offer speedier healing and symptom relief.

   –If you are not especially bothered by symptoms or high outbreak frequency, you may still wish to consider taking an oral antiviral medicine on a short-term but continuous basis to reduce the frequency of episodes during special occasions— e.g., new relationships, vacations, new jobs, or, if appropriate for you, periods of high stress.

   –If you decide that your type of genital herpes does not call for treatment, then do not take treatment. You need not use ineffective medicines or change your lifestyle or alter your diet or your own pattern of living to try to get herpes to go away. There are safe treatments that will make herpes outbreaks disappear more quickly and come back less frequently. After the primary episode is over, though, some people may not require treatment. Many alternative suggestions from health food stores and well-intentioned friends do not directly address the problem you are facing. Be careful to avoid using medications incorrectly or taking medications that are unproven.

5. Be realistic. Researching herpes for the sake of knowledge and in order to regain control over your own life is a goal to be applauded. You will not, however, find a cure by frantically reading all the latest literature. Hoping for a cure is fine. It is critical that a cure, an effective method of prevention, and improved treatment be found. For now, establish an easy method for keeping up with the latest in herpes research so that good treatments come to your attention. There have been major advances in therapy of herpes in the past ten years. There has even been a Nobel prize given to Gertrude Belle Elion and George Herbert Hitchings from Burroughs Wellcome for discoveries in this area. Therapy is safe and effective. As of today, ideas for scientifically sound cures are not being tested in clinical trials. Yet, for the first time, scientists are now discussing how they might approach the cure of herpes.

6. Avoid unproven promises of cure. Even if you choose alternative methods of therapy, be careful to obtain standard therapy as well. Be selective in choosing either a standard or an alternative therapy. Be wary of people selling snake oil from expensive clinics in foreign countries promising cures for large sums of money.

7. If your anger is a problem for you, seek and find logical and acceptable answers to your questions. Participate actively in finding those answers, and get herpes into perspective. *Herpes is not you.* It is, however, a reality in your life. If you are pregnant, make sure that the person scheduled to follow your pregnancy and help you deliver your baby knows what to do when the time comes. If you are concerned about cervical cancer, have yearly Pap tests and remember that the risk is low. If you are concerned about spreading herpes, keep in mind that the caring and educated person with herpes who tries to avoid transmitting herpes generally does so with a great deal of success. Find an appropriate person to talk to about herpes—a health care practitioner, another person with herpes you find at a self-help group, or a knowledgeable and trusted friend.

8. If you believe that your feelings or symptoms fit the category

"clinical depression," seek assistance. Call your own doctor or a crisis hotline or go to an emergency room of a hospital. Counseling can also be of great assistance to anyone whose life is being significantly disrupted by herpes. A good counselor can help people to face their fears and help people who are stuck feeling like victims to get unstuck. A counselor can be a very valuable resource when you are considering whether or how to tell your new partner that you have herpes.

9. Avoid blaming someone else or yourself for your herpes. Our society is all too often blame-oriented, and herpes transmission becomes the focus of blame in some situations. Of course, sometimes it is necessary to fix blame—for example, if genital herpes results from rape or some other malicious intent. But if a mutually consenting relationship led to the transmission of genital herpes, it is rarely useful to blame your partner. Focusing on blaming someone else prevents you from healing yourself mentally and getting on with your life. Blaming yourself serves no useful purpose either. People run special risks of getting stuck when it comes to blame. To move on with the important things in your life, to make sure you obtain whatever new information you may need to help you with future decisions, you will almost always be better off putting the blame issues behind you as soon as you can.

10. When you are ready, get on with your life. You can live a normal and healthy life—whatever that is for you—and also have genital herpes. You need not feel like a victim. Promise yourself you won't.

11. Think about how you are keeping the matter of your herpes private. Are you merely maintaining your privacy or are you hiding your darkest secret? If herpes is your big secret, commit yourself to putting it into better perspective. You can keep herpes a private matter, but make certain you have someone you can discuss your feelings with. You can reach out to someone else and also keep herpes a private matter if you confide in a friend or a health care professional with whom you have established a good relationship. You can keep herpes private while getting rid of the trap of keeping it a secret.

Herpes—a deep, dark secret or simply a private matter?

If all the people you know knew you had herpes, how would your life change? What if all people with herpes were named in a list in the newspaper each day and kept on a public list somewhere? For many people I know, this idea causes fear in the pit of the stomach. In our society, we often choose to keep these things private. It is usually to your advantage to avoid making your herpes the subject of others' gossip. Herpes can be a juicy story, and, generally, you are best off not becoming the subject. For the sake of privacy, then, you may not wish to mention your herpes casually or socially. It is simply not anyone else's business, unless you plan to have sexual contact with that person.

On the other hand, as far-fetched as it may seem, what if everyone with genital herpes wore a button saying "I have genital herpes." One of every four or five people would be wearing the button. People would have to come to terms with herpes and put it in perspective. Everyone would have to deal with the matter with many of their friends and family members. Any stereotypes people might have about herpes would quickly fade away. The feeling that you are alone with this infection would quickly disappear. Of course, for now, no one is wearing this button. You should not be the first, either. I am not trying to start a new button revolution; nor am I suggesting that the private matter of having herpes is not, indeed, private.

Imagine yourself wearing this herpes button, though, and ask yourself: "Would my life be improved, ruined, or unchanged by this button, if I and all other people with herpes were wearing one?" If your life would be unchanged, then privacy is just that—privacy. Many people with herpes, though, become trapped by the secrecy they impose upon themselves. You may wish to determine just how much your secret is helping you or hurting you. Ask yourself, is keeping the secret taking a significant investment of mental energy each day? How important is this secret?

In general, it is probably still wise to avoid discussions about your herpes with casual friends and acquaintances, as long as you are in comfortable control of the privacy process. It is just as important, however, to share your feelings with at least one person. Consider sharing the facts and possibly also your feelings about your herpes in the following circumstances:

1. Share information if sharing it will help you in some important way. For example, you must tell your doctor so that he or she can make sure you have been properly diagnosed as having herpes and do not have any other illness or infection requiring treatment. Then he or she can help you with treatment or counseling. Or tell members of a self-help group with whom you share similar personal experiences. You may also choose to share the information with a close friend. Sharing your feelings is a personal decision. Many people choose never to tell friends. They diminish the risks inherent in "going public." In making that choice, however, they also lose an important opportunity for sharing feelings. In general, it is good advice to try your best to find at least one person with whom you can let out your feelings and fears. Keep yourself connected with the world and try not to let the secret itself take over your control of having herpes.

2. When you choose to tell a friend with whom you have no sexual intimacy or plans for sexual intimacy, you may wish to consider in advance who might be the right person. Casual acquaintances are generally unwise choices here, unless you have decided to tell everyone. Many people talk casually and openly about herpes, though, and doing this absolutely prevents the secret itself from becoming a burden. When you do discuss herpes, no matter with whom, you have every right to ask for confidentiality. In the case of your doctor or health care professional, he or she is sworn to an oath of secrecy, of course. In the case of a nonprofessional, choose someone who you feel confident will respect your privacy. Explain to this friend that you want to avoid pity. The last thing you need is someone to feel sorry for you; the right friend will not pity you, but rather will help you to avoid self-pity. If you feel that you would benefit from having someone close to talk to about herpes, search out an equal who will not use the information to feel superior but will offer personal advice and criticism. A good friend has

confidence in your own abilities to resolve your own problems. He or she is willing to act as a nonjudgmental sounding board and to stand behind you as you solve your own dilemma. A good friend does not need to take over and fix your problem for you, although he or she may offer information about available resources and may offer another perspective about how to look at your situation. You may gain a great deal from using the mental energy and resources acquired from friendship as a springboard to getting on with your life.

3. You will also want to share the facts about your herpes if sharing the information will help someone else in some important way. For example, tell your present and future sexual partners, a friend who has herpes, etc. Sort out your thoughts about telling sexual partners.

Should I tell my new sexual partner that I have herpes?

This is a very delicate question that no third person outside the relationship can answer. Through my experience of talking with people who have herpes, I have heard many opinions expressed. Because of the natural tendency to moralize when dealing with a difficult subject like this, many answers are inadequate. Rather than offer you yet another set of prejudices, I will draw some analogies and ask some questions based on patients' concerns. For a person making her or his own decision about whether to discuss herpes, past experience, advice from others, and intuition may all be helpful.

We live in an age of informed consent. Basic medical ethics and the courts have decided that the physician must inform the patient about inherent risks from drugs or from surgery. Even if I, as a physician, believe the chances of side effects occurring from a certain drug in any one individual to be very small, I am obligated to discuss them in order to give the person the opportunity to decide. Sharing the information relieves me of the responsibility I would have held had I not explained the side effects. I am still held responsible to uphold my duty to prevent those side effects, if possible. My responsibilities fit the situation, in that I am responsible for my actions but not guilty of withholding the truth.

As a physician trained to know, or at least expected to know, about side effects, I can easily appreciate that the chances of bad things happening to a particular person are very low. I may choose to avoid discussing all the details, thinking I can avoid causing needless concern in a patient unlikely to experience particular side effects. I thus save the patient some anxiety and save myself time and the difficulty of explaining. Indeed, for practical reasons, many physicians do this daily. The physician chooses which side effects to discuss on the basis of their severity and their likelihood of occurrence as well as on the basis of the individual physician's ease with the patient and how well he or she understands the side effects. Many other factors play a role. For example, how busy is the office? How many times has the same thing been said? How well does the physician believe the patient will understand the information? Will the patient be frightened?

When discussing your herpes with your partner, you have a relationship that closely parallels that of the doctor and the patient. There appear to be many legal parallels as well. You hold information in your head about yourself that may influence how your partner will feel or act. You have power over your partner, in the sense that knowledge is power. If you avoid sharing the information, you create an unequal balance in your relationship. Any secret one partner withholds from the other changes that delicate balance.

On the other hand, your relationship may not be at the stage where you wish to establish that balance or equality. If you are involved in a casual relationship, you may feel that your partner is not close enough to share such information with. The risk of transmitting herpes during one encounter in an inactive phase is certainly quite low. Furthermore, any two people in a casual encounter take certain risks of transmitting and receiving infections. If you have a short-term encounter, you generally know that you are taking risks. (Of course, because of the risks of other sexually transmitted diseases, especially human immunodeficiency virus (HIV) infection, you are well advised to avoid casual sexual encounters altogether, whether or not you have herpes.)

Your decision about whether or not to tell is a personal one. It may also be partly based on personal experience. For example, were you told about the risks when you contracted herpes? Could you have been? Have you passed herpes on to anyone before? You may decide to withhold the information because it is difficult to tell or because you are a shy or private person. You may decide to tell because of your conscience or your moral convictions; it may be easier for you to tell than not to tell. It is a matter of personal integrity; your conscience must compare your right to privacy with your partner's right to informed consent. Choosing to tell is, in some circumstances, the more difficult path to choose. Sometimes telling may seem unnecessary. Discussing herpes before having sex may give herpes unwarranted status, especially if you feel in physical control of your infection. Unfortunately, the facts about asymptomatic transmission of herpes do not support the notion that a person with clear symptoms can completely control or prevent transmission. Some people note that even though most people have oral herpes, the average person with cold sores does not talk about cold sores before kissing or having oral-genital contact. If a person knows that there is a risk, however small, what should be told and what should not be told? Should the person who had one episode of genital herpes five years ago discuss herpes before each new sexual encounter? If not, where should the line be drawn? Should a person not discuss oral sores that have recurred monthly since he or she was kissed as a child, because they came from his or her mother and not a lover?

If you wish to tell your partner everything, you could say the following: "By the way, I get recurrences of herpes on my mouth, so when I have a sore we will have to avoid kissing and oral sex," or "I get recurrences of herpes on my genitals, so when I have a sore we will have to avoid genital sex, and we should probably be considering safer sex practices, anyway." If instead of genital herpes, you had just found out that you were a carrier of human immunodeficiency virus or hepatitis B virus, how would this change your discussion policy? Is it the relative mildness of herpes that seems to make discussion less necessary? People who have hepatitis B or human immunodeficiency virus have these discussions every day. There are steps to take to prevent transmission, and both partners need to share openly for them to be optimally effective. For example, the hepatitis B carrier's partner needs to be vaccinated, and until protective antibody is present, safer sex precautions need to be practiced. It is always easier to prevent transmission and deal with issues when both people share equally in the access to information. Regardless of the situation, you owe it to your current or future partner, your current or future relationship, and, most of all, to yourself, to learn the art of discussing herpes.

I routinely ask people, "How does herpes affect your life?" Answers to this question almost universally lie not within the realm of the physical ailment itself—i.e., the pain of an outbreak or the need for quicker healing of sores. More than anything else in the world, people who come to see me with herpes want to avoid transmitting herpes to their partner—current or future. They also want to know that their partner will accept them—herpes and all. When it comes to telling your partner about herpes, there are two choices:

1. You might choose not to discuss herpes with your partner.
Some people are just not willing to go through the process of discussing herpes. They cope with their unwillingness to discuss herpes by just not having the discussion. They may carefully avoid contact during active phases of infection and use safer sexual practices. These methods of avoiding transmission, however, do not make the herpes discussion unnecessary. In fact, this route is the most dangerous option for both partners. It is dangerous for the secret-keeper because it keeps that person in hiding and heightens personal vulnerability in the relationship. People who have taken this option may find themselves doing things they would not ordinarily do, such as sometimes breaking off relationships before they get too close, in order to avoid the discussion. Once the secret is set in motion and sexual contact has taken place, it may seem harder with each passing encounter to have the discussion. The more you like the other person, the more you may subconsciously want to break off the relationship so that you do not need to find out if the person will really reject you. Or you may find yourself having only casual encounters that seem to call for no discussion—an especially dangerous choice in the age of AIDS and one that works against the process of self-acceptance.

For some people, keeping the secret means sharing it with no partner—ever. But this leaves only one of two options. Either they have sexual relationships without talking about herpes, or they avoid sexual relationships in order to dodge the issue entirely. Neither choice is healthy. It is possible to choose celibacy from a positive position of strength—a personal choice arrived at by a choosy person making a lifestyle decision. However, most people I have met who choose celibacy after herpes do not do so from a position of strength. If the choice is made because of the herpes secret, it is not a simple personal choice but rather a new place to get stuck where most would probably rather not be. Celibacy, of course, causes no danger to any partner and brings the entire burden upon oneself. It may seem for a while as if this is almost appropriate. People sometimes say, "I have no one to blame but myself." Celibacy for a short period of time is very common for people with herpes who have an adjustment period while getting to know their herpes and getting comfortable with the idea of telling. A substantial minority of patients choose celibacy for prolonged periods.

It is OK to reestablish relationships after acquiring herpes. If you find it easier to "fold" when given the chance of a new relationship, then you may be making that decision out of a position of weakness rather than strength. Relationships and lovers are not for everyone. This society has become more accepting of people who choose celibacy or avoidance of romance. But if you were going to choose this route out of strength, why did you not choose it earlier?

If you believe that your celibacy arises from a reaction to your having herpes and not from a personal, assertive choice, and if it continues for a long time, I strongly recommend that you sit down with a professional counselor and work through these issues. You may want to begin this discussion with your doctor, depending on how comfortable you are with him or her. You owe it to yourself to discuss this. Sometimes just talking about it can be very frightening, but talking about it is also very freeing, since you have the opportunity to say out loud how you feel and what the factors are that are keeping you stuck. One discussion may not be enough, and it does not always go exactly the way you hoped. Do not hesitate to get good counseling if you feel you need it. Every person deserves and needs the opportunity to work out feelings and vulnerabilities openly and honestly.

Herpes is sometimes the straw that broke the camel's back. People who get herpes sometimes find that their interpersonal relationships haven't been going the way they wished anyway and that herpes is just one very visible manifestation of that. Herpes may be the opportunity for you to come to grips with your situation and to start some counseling or whatever is required to sort out whatever got you there in the first place. If you have chosen celibacy, be sure that you really want to be there before you just accept it as inevitable. It isn't.

One alternative to celibacy is simply to avoid the topic and to have relationships—casual or long-term—as if herpes were not an issue. This is potentially the worst of all possible traps, however. Some people feel justified in not telling because they feel that using chronic oral antiviral medication to suppress herpes and/or safer sex practices makes the discussion unnecessary. I have seen couples who have been together for ten years suddenly lose the secret at the time of delivery of a fourth child because an active outbreak at delivery required cesarean section. In general, the more someone means to you, the more you will want them to know about your herpes. Closeness, alone, however, does not make it possible to have the discussion. The longer a person keeps their herpes secret, the harder it is to reveal.

There is one more very practical reason to tell your partner—the legal one. Litigation is a fact of life these days, especially in the United States and Canada. It is becoming more clear that transmission of herpes can be the subject of a successful lawsuit, especially if the herpes secret has been kept. Keeping the secret is understandable, but it is not at all advisable. I am not a lawyer, but I understand that if transmission can be proved (this is often extremely difficult to do based on the facts of a case), the remaining 99 percent of the litigation-for-herpes issue is the question of how well informed the partner was (assuming that the original person with herpes was aware of the diagnosis).

Most people who choose the path of secrecy are just not willing to make themselves vulnerable. Some feel that they are waiting for just the right moment—for example, the moment when the relationship becomes based on mutual trust. But a policy of not telling while sharing sexual intimacy may be interpreted retroactively by a partner as a breach of trust. A partner's willingness to be understanding is put at more risk with each passing day of silence on the topic of herpes. The best advice for someone stuck holding the secret is to bite the bullet and have the discussion. Eventually, if the relationship is worth having, the discussion has to be held. Do not interpret this advice, though, as a guilt-trip by the herpes doctor. If you cannot bring yourself to bite this bullet, but you would like to, you can get help from a relationship or family counselor, for example.

2. You might choose to discuss herpes with your partner.
If you have chosen to discuss your herpes, you have chosen a very honorable path. This task can be difficult. Choosing to do it shows your honesty and the concern you feel for your partner. It shows that you care so much about your relationship that you are willing to expose your own vulnerability. You deserve to be rewarded for having overcome whatever personal fear has been keeping you stuck. Getting unstuck feels great and is a reward in and of itself, even if your fears are realized and the conversation does not go your way. Facing a fear and growing from it helps to make one courageous. It helps to remove a victim label, if there is one.

One thing is for certain—you do not owe anyone an apology for having herpes. Besides learning that you have herpes, your partner also finds out other things about you when you tell him or her about your herpes infection. He or she finds out that you are concerned about your own sexual health and the sexual health of your partner and that you have taken the trouble to know and understand what safer sexual practices really mean. By now, you have probably made sure that you do not have other sexually transmitted infections or, if you do, that you have learned what they are and how to avoid transmitting them.

If your partner is also honest and sensitive and caring, he or she will, at the very least, respect what you have done and agree to let you decide with whom you will choose to share your secret. There is absolutely no excuse for anyone to discuss your secret with another party without your express permission. You should ask for and receive the promise to have your secret kept. If your partner does not make that promise or breaks it, perhaps you should have chosen someone else anyway and should be more selective next time. But do not give up. Not every partner will choose to continue to develop a sexual relationship. This discussion is about informed consent: some people will choose not to accept a risk. Ironically, those people may be increasing rather than reducing their risk of acquiring herpes. Nevertheless, the decision is theirs. For some, the herpes discussion is just the excuse they needed to get out of a relationship they were not too sure of to begin with. Others will want to have time to adjust or think about what you have said or learn more. Welcome your thoughtful partner's desire for further medical information. Honest understanding with acceptance is what you seek. Many people will turn ahead the calendar in their own mind to picture themselves in relationship with you several months ahead. If that mental picture is mutually loving and nurturing—i.e., if your partner pictures being lovers with you for a while to come—then, chances are, your partner will find out what he or she needs to know about herpes, take appropriate precautions, and proceed with the relationship. If your lover-to-be looks in the crystal ball only to see himself or herself with another partner, there is a good chance that the herpes discussion will provide the correct time for that change to take place. It is unusual for genital herpes to come permanently between partners in an otherwise sound and mutually beneficial relationship that is committed to growth. Hang on for that one, since that is the one worth having, anyway. In fact, many people with herpes use this discussion opportunity to their advantage. A herpes discussion is a very good way of finding committed partners early in a relationship. If you can have this discussion in a clear and thoughtful manner, without apology and without feeling too vulnerable, you can begin to take very positive and assertive control over your life. Use herpes discussions to your advantage to raise your self-esteem rather than give it away. If you take control of this and do not place your self-esteem or happiness into the lap of your discussion partner, you will find the experience uplifting.

So what should I do if my partner told me about his or her herpes after we established a sexual relationship? Does that mean my partner is dishonest?

If you are the partner who has not been told, if may help to keep in mind that this struggle is difficult for everyone with herpes. In the short term, it is definitely easier not to tell. For some people, getting over this hurdle is extremely difficult or even overwhelmingly frightening. If your partner knew about her or his herpes and did not tell you, he or she was probably wanting to tell you more than anything. There is often a very honest person behind the veil of herpes secrecy—usually a person whose vulnerability in the area of sexuality and relationships is very high. It is understandable to feel wronged if your partner has not told you about herpes. Take a moment before reacting severely to this mistake, however. People with vulnerabilities make mistakes. The fact that you have been told after sexual intimacy has begun does not take away your own future choices. If your relationship is otherwise strong, you and your partner can use this experience to strengthen your bond with each other and to learn more about each other and each other's frailties. Taking this as an opportunity to score a point or to win something against your partner would not help your relationship or help you to move forward in your own life.

How should I tell my sexual partner?

There is a lot of advice around, published and unpublished, about herpes discussions. Generally, it is agreed that herpes should be put into perspective, not made more or less of than it is. Remember that your own overall feeling about this infection will come through strongly when you tell your lover-to-be. Avoid preparing for the discussion by painting a picture of impending doom. Stay away from a tone or words that suggest "Sit down—I have something horrible to tell you" or "Prepare yourself." Your role is simply to inform. Tell your partner everything you know about herpes—what it is, how you know you have it, how you avoid transmitting it, what asymptomatic shedding is, how you have handled telling people before, etc. You may wish to practice role-playing first with a friend or counselor.

Tell your partner early but not too early. Once you have established mutual trust and realize you want to have a sexual relationship with this person, then talk about herpes before you are physically involved. The subject of herpes has a powerful way of curbing spontaneity or spoiling the moment. Thought and sexual arousal are not well-suited partners. Plan the moment. Whether you choose a long walk or a dinner is not important, but the absence of sexual contact is. The discussion should take place where sexual contact is unlikely to follow the discussion. To truly provide informed consent to your partner, you will want to give him or her a day or so to think about it. More time may be required if your partner wants to read about herpes or talk to his or her own health care provider. You must be comfortable with the knowledge you possess, since you must serve as an initial source of information. Avoid using your knowledge to one-up or one-down the person you are talking with. Instead, educate your partner on an equal basis—make it a shared experience. Do your best to stay in control of the situation. You have some medical facts to discuss and some plans for avoiding transmission. You will want to tell your partner that this is something he or she is being entrusted with because you feel that the relationship is worthy of it and you sense that sexual involvement may soon develop.

Clarity, honesty and assertiveness without apology are the keys to discussing herpes with a new sexual partner-to-be. Talking about herpes with a new partner can be the most difficult part of having herpes. You are putting your vulnerability on the line to protect your partner's welfare and make your relationship honest and open. These are very honorable things to do and you should congratulate yourself for having the courage. Having the discussion raises you from the status of victim to the status of honest, concerned partner. Clarity, honesty, and assertiveness without apology are useful qualities when talking with the boss at work. To maintain these qualities when talking about your sexuality and showing your vulnerability in a relationship with someone you don't yet know well can be a major challenge.

Expect some expression of fear from your partner. Acceptance without fear could mean that your partner knows about herpes already or else that he or she is not dealing with the subject.

Expressed fears can be dealt with and placed into perspective; you should do your best to encourage your new partner to use clarity, honesty, and assertiveness without apology also. You will want to avoid creating any unclear or unequal situation between you or manipulating your partner with guilt or emotional traps—just as you will want to avoid having your partner place you in an emotional trap. Most people will not get up and run from a relationship because of herpes. Remember that herpes is not you, any more than the acne on your back is you or the bump on your nose is you. You need not apologize for having herpes—not to yourself *or* to your partner—and you certainly do not need to apologize for talking about it. If you find it especially difficult to talk about herpes in the situation of a casual encounter, you might be advised to opt for avoiding casual relationships or else telling anyway. Going ahead with a casual relationship and avoiding the subject of herpes can be tempting. Entering into a secret situation with a lover, however, is unwise. By now, it should be obvious that I feel you have a moral responsibility to yourself and to your partner to have this discussion.

What about after I've told my partner-to-be?

After you've told your partner, there are more potential traps to look out for. After you've talked about your herpes, you will want to remember to keep your self-esteem and your self-confidence under your own control. It is pleasant, of course, when your partner-to-be accepts you with your herpes and all. But be careful not to tie your happiness to whether she or he responds positively. If you did your job well in this discussion and your partner-to-be stopped the relationship, mourn the loss of the possible relationship. Do that only for a short time, though, and then move on. Imagine what would have happened if you had been in this relationship for a long time and then developed multiple sclerosis, or your oldest child was arrested for shoplifting, or any other crisis came up in your life. Someone who leaves a relationship for herpes alone was very likely not fully committed in the first place. Despite how vulnerable you may feel, the short-term pain or awkwardness will be a positive investment in your own future.

You deserve a partner who sees your herpes as simply a detail that needs attention.

Whether your partner responds well to your discussion or not, know that you have done the right thing. To entrust your self-esteem to someone who you are just getting to know is not advisable—even if it feels good for the moment and especially if it feels bad.

What is a self-help group?

Since the dawn of history, people with similar problems and related goals have shared them for mutual benefit. This special kind of community has proven useful for everything from coping with recurring genital sores to fighting world wars. People with herpes may wish to come together for a number of different reasons:

Emotional Support
- participating in group discussions
- sharing similar experiences
- receiving group support
- venting anger in a sympathetic forum
- allaying your own fears by relating them to others

Information Transfer
- making accurate information available to everyone
- keeping abreast of changes in the field

Political Forum
- working to influence government decisions on, for example, education, prevention, treatment, and spending of health-care dollars

Charitable Support
- fund raising
- organizing direct monetary support of clinical facilities and herpes hotlines
- supporting basic and clinical research
- training personnel to meet future needs

In deciding how to organize a self-help group, you first need to set goals. Which reasons have brought you together? If emotional support is the only goal, then a local support group is the only necessity. First check to see if a group already exists in your community. You may call local health resource centers, women's health centers, sexually transmitted diseases clinics, public health authorities, or a local herpes clinic, if there is one in your area. The national organizations listed in appendix 1 may be able to refer you to a local chapter if you live in North America. In any group, it is important that some or all of the members be well informed.

If you want to work for goals other than emotional support, it is helpful to join a national organization, if your country has one.

What's good about herpes?

The diagnosis of herpes is a fork in the road. It is an unexpected, uninvited, and unwanted intruder into your life. It comes suddenly and strikes in subtle ways. Yet there is always potential in crisis. If nothing else, herpes is a learning experience: most people who get herpes learn more about biology, medicine, pharmacology, nutrition, and personal communication in the few months following diagnosis than they had learned in their entire lives. A herpes crisis is an opportunity to get to know yourself.

Sexual freedom without a care is over. The disadvantages to this are clear. Herpes, however, promotes honest and open discussion early in relationships. The concern herpes raises in people about their sexual habits has probably prevented thousands of cases of other sexually transmitted infections, because genital herpes forces a change in personal lifestyle. Dr. Suzanne Kroon, of Copenhagen, Denmark, describes this as herpes-induced "quality control." You can use herpes to help yourself be selective in the partner selection process. It provides an opportunity to face your vulnerability and take control.

In some cases, the openness triggered by the need to talk about herpes improve the quality of relationships. Establishing communication about herpes makes it easier for people to discuss serious personal concerns as well. Because of the stress introduced into the relationship by herpes, other problems may be brought forward. You would often have had to work through these problems eventually. If your partner picks your herpes as a reason to leave, it may be for the best—as long as it was not based on medical misunderstanding, which can be corrected. In everyone's life at some point, something goes wrong. You might get injured in a car accident or get very sick. If your partner leaves on account of your herpes, imagine what would have happened had you been put into a wheelchair or scarred by a fire. Eventually you will die. Possibly you've found the worm in the apple before you bit too deeply.

Herpes forces people to learn about themselves and about herpes and to talk about themselves with others. For people who have never been able to talk about intimate feelings and personal matters, herpes can be a springboard. Clarity and honesty and assertiveness without apology are traits that everyone should have. Herpes may be the tool that helps you achieve them, and it may also make you more sensitive to the needs of others who face similar decisions.

People who know definitely that they have herpes have a distinct advantage over people who have it and do not know: they are able to distinguish active from latent phases and can avoid infecting others. People who know they have herpes, take care to avoid active phases of infection, and use safer sex practices and other means of reducing transmission risks, are better equipped to avoid transmitting herpes than those who feel they do not have it. People who think they do not have herpes may be right or wrong.

Herpes is a big change for some people and a small change for others. There are some obvious bad points to be confronted and dealt with. There are also changes for the good. Get over the tough parts by facing them directly: learn the coping methods, be aware of new developments, and, for now, accept the change and the challenge to normalize your life in the face of adversity. Herpes will probably affect you only once in a while. You have a virus for life, but you do not have a disease for life.

9

Some Special Problems

Homosexuals are really (physiologically) like heterosexuals!
(Catholics are, physiologically, like Protestants; Jews are,
physiologically, like Moslems.) Indeed they are. But the plea
for accepting a minority because it resembles the majority is,
in effect, a denial of the minority's right to be different.

—THOMAS SZASZ
Sex by Prescription

Herpes and the homosexual male

Homosexual men used to have a much higher risk than heterosexual men of contracting sexually transmitted infections. Because of AIDS, this risk has been substantially reduced, through a decrease in the numbers of sexual partners and the adoption of safer sex techniques. Penile sores in homosexuals are the same as penile sores in heterosexuals. Since herpes simplex virus tends to cause infection where it is inoculated, anal intercourse can result in inoculation of virus to the anus. Thus, anal herpes is common among homosexual men. *Internal* infection of the anus is rare in the absence of anal intercourse, although both women and heterosexual men commonly experience *external*, or perianal, infection.

Inflammation of the anus is called *proctitis*. Many different infectious agents, including gonorrhea, Chlamydia, and syphilis, can cause proctitis. Noninfectious causes include sexual intercourse (which can cause tearing or abrasion of anal tissue) and ulcerative colitis. Generally, although not always, herpes proctitis results from a primary herpes infection of the rectum. Whereas recurrent herpes in this area tends to be mild and external (like recurrent herpes anywhere else), primary herpes proctitis may result in mul-

193

tiple discomforts during the initial episode. Rectal pain is very common. *Tenesmus,* or an urgent feeling of needing to pass stool whether stool is present or not, is universal. A discharge from the rectum is also common. This discharge may be bloody. Most people become somewhat constipated, and itching may be disturbing. Pains of the low back, buttocks, and thigh are often present. Such pains may also accompany genital herpes without proctitis. They are called *sacral paresthesias.* Nearly half of affected men have difficulty passing urine during this primary episode. Other problems resulting from inflammation of nerves, such as temporary impotence, occur less often. Lesions may be seen externally around the anus or may be present only internally. Fever and swollen glands in the groin are also common. The overwhelming majority of men have positive virus cultures from the rectum. After one to six weeks, the symptoms clear. This infection parallels cervical infection of women in being both internal and external, while recurrent herpes is almost exclusively external.

If I am female and homosexual, can I get herpes?

Yes. The risk of acquiring genital herpes type 2 is slightly less for heterosexual women, because there is less genital-to-genital contact, the usual route of type 2 transmission. However, transmission of type 2 herpes between partners using shared sex objects or hands is definitely possible. The risk of acquiring type 1 genital herpes is slightly increased because of increased oral-to-genital contact. Because the main methods of transmission are oral-to-oral and oral-to-genital, there is a greater theoretical chance of acquiring herpes simplex virus type 1. Otherwise, the risks and outcome of a herpes infection are identical in homosexual and heterosexual women.

Are herpes and AIDS related?

Like genital herpes, *acquired immune deficiency syndrome* (AIDS) is most often sexually transmitted. Herpes simplex virus grows inside skin or epithelial cells, which then form a genital sore and, in turn, cause infection in a sexual partner by direct sore-to-skin contact. By contrast, the *human immunodeficiency virus* (HIV), the virus that causes AIDS, hides inside the immune cells. Some of these cells circulate in the blood, from where they are sent to fight infections. Immune cells are also sent to the skin surface to fight off infections and other intruders. Some of these cells spill into the semen of men with HIV. Others travel to the skin and mucosal surfaces to lead the fight against infections such as herpes and other sexually transmitted diseases. When the infected cells from the body fluids of one person spend time in direct contact with the healthy immune cells of a susceptible partner, a new infection takes place. AIDS threatens heterosexuals and homosexuals. People with AIDS lose the part of the immune system infected with HIV known as the cellular immune system. The cells that make up this component of the immune system are the lymphocytes.

When infected with HIV, the lymphocytes eventually die and so are not available to fight off infection. As a result, people with AIDS may fall victim to infections or tumors. Specifically, tumors such as *Kaposi's sarcoma* and *lymphoma* are found. Very unusual infections that are not seen in people with normal immunity are also encountered, such as PCP (*Pneumocystis carinii pneumonia*) and a host of other infections.

So what does all of this have to do with genital herpes? HIV and herpes simplex are both sexually transmitted, but the methods of cellular transmission are very different: one moves from cell to cell by direct contact with skin; the other moves from cell to cell by direct contact with immune cells contained in body fluids and mucosal surfaces. Yet herpes and AIDS have a lot in common. The first AIDS patients ever described were suffering from unusually severe and difficult herpes infections that failed to recover in the normal time. When the chief immune cells used to fight herpes are wiped out by AIDS, herpes becomes a bigger problem than when the immune system is intact. When herpes affects someone with inadequate immunity, many complications can occur. The sores may not heal spontaneously, as they normally would, and may develop into larger and more extensive ulcers. Parallels exist with the newborn herpes syndrome, where, because of immature immunity, the virus may spread to internal organs. Herpes is highly treatable under these conditions; intravenous or oral acyclovir (Zovirax), valacyclovir (Valtrex) or famciclovir (Famvir) generally stop progression of the virus. But because AIDS continues to suppress immunity, herpes infections may recur or progress without therapy. People with AIDS and others whose immunity is severely compromised, as it is in certain cancers or after transplantation, may find that antiviral treatments taken in appropriate doses stops working. This can result from true antiviral resistance, in which the virus adapts to the drug and becomes immune to treatment. To date, significant antiviral resistance has only been consistently found in people with compromised immunity. Generally, the breakthrough mild outbreaks seen in people with normal immunity are not truly resistant to treatment. Where true antiviral resistance does occur, therapy must be switched temporarily to an alternative drug such as foscarnet or cidofovir.

During a herpes infection, the body calls into action all of its defenses. One of its key soldiers is a set of immune cells called CD4 or T4 *lymphocytes*, which boost the positive side of the immune system. The CD4 cells are one of the most effective fighters we have against herpes. They are the targets of HIV, which depletes them, thereby disrupting immunity and leading to AIDS. During a herpes outbreak, these immune soldier cells are right at the surface of the skin or mucus membrane, fighting against herpes. While the cells are busy clearing up the herpes infection, they sit like targets for HIV right at the body surface. Having sex at that moment with a partner who has HIV eases transmission of the virus. It is a bit like luring the soldiers out of the fort for an ambush. When the CD4 lymphocytes are inside the fort (inside the blood circulation), HIV needs to make a deeper entry to accomplish its goal of infection. Even when the situation is perfect for HIV transmission, proper use of safer sex practices is very effective at minimizing the risk of transmission. Furthermore, I believe (based solely on personal impressions, without sound epidemiological data to back me up) that many people with herpes who inform themselves about herpes actually reduce their risk of getting *all* sexually transmitted diseases, including herpes, AIDS, Chlamydia, gonorrhea, and hepatitis B, by becoming more careful in choosing sexual partners, minimizing casual relationships, and adopting safer sex practices when they enter into new relationships.

Can herpes kill?

Yes, herpes can kill, but it does so only very rarely. Regular skin-type herpes does not suddenly go wild and cause serious physical illness. Herpes can kill only under very specific circumstances: the newborn baby whose immune system has not matured; the adult who, for reasons we do not understand, develops herpes encephalitis, a brain infection; or the person whose immune system fails, resulting in rampant and widespread herpes. If you have herpes somewhere on your skin—whether on your lip, your genitals, or your toe—herpes is not likely to harm you physically now or in the future.

Will I have herpes for as long as I live?

Yes—and no. As far as we know, once latent infection has been established in the ganglion (which usually occurs before you even realize you have herpes), the latent state persists for life. Active infection does not persist, however. Active phases of infection occur sporadically, when the herpes reactivates. Some people with a recurrent herpes infection are bothered less frequently after the first several years. Others note that their recurrence pattern just keeps going with no change. A high frequency pattern that persists can be quite distressing; in this case, it may be beneficial to use drugs to suppress outbreaks. Why herpes reactivations persist at high frequency in some people is not understood.

For some people with herpes, a time comes when recurrences decrease in frequency. There are no known explanations for why this happens. If the body's immune system figures out new tricks to kill the virus, scientists have so far been unable to detect them. Another possibility is that virus may be reactivated in many of the ganglionic nerve cells affected by latent herpes. Once the infection has been reactivated in one cell, that cell probably dies, leaving the person with fewer total affected cells with each recurrence. Nobody knows the actual process. If this phenomenon could be understood and reproduced with a drug, the drug's patent would be an excellent one to hold. The virus itself, however, does not actually burn out in the ganglion. Even without recurrences, if something happens to suddenly alter the immune system (for example, leukemia or AIDS), the latent virus will once again reactivate. Clinically active recurrences, though, change their patterns all the time. Herpes can slow down for awhile, suddenly get more frequent, and slow down again. This is one of the key reasons why carefully controlled, double-blind, clinical trials are required to substantiate the efficacy of new treatments for herpes, even where honest people swear by the benefits of one or another treatment.

Herpes and eczema

Skin diseases such as eczema that cause multiple breaks in the integrity of the skin barrier may, in unusual circumstances, predispose people to more severe herpes simplex infections. Under these circumstances, during primary herpes—oral or genital—the virus can work its way into every available skin tear caused by eczema. This syndrome is called *eczema herpeticum* or *Kaposi's varicelliform eruption*. Generally, lesions heal after about six weeks. Although recurrent outbreaks of eczema herpeticum can be problematic, they, like recurrent herpes in people who do not have eczema, are usually milder than primary outbreaks because of general immunity against herpes. Eczema does not really diminish the overall immune response that much. The immune problem here seems to be mainly an interruption of normal mechanical skin barriers. Since eczema can occur anywhere but especially likes the scalp and hands, herpes infections occur in places that are unusual for herpes.

People with significant eczema who develop primary herpes should be extremely careful to avoid self-inoculation. If the problem is severe, they may also wish to use antiviral medication. Properly used, antiviral agents markedly reduce the duration and limit the complications of eczema herpeticum.

Occupational herpes hazards: Can I get herpes at work?

The answer depends on the type of work you do. If your only contact with people on the job is shaking hands, you are at very low risk of contracting herpes at work. If you sell kisses at carnivals, your chances increase quite a bit. If you sell kisses on the street your chances become close to 100 percent. Many other occupations involve close person-to-person contact. One example used to be dentistry. Each dentist sees many people every day and, over time, has his or her hands in thousands of mouths. Before AIDS, it was common for dentists to work without wearing gloves and to wash their hands very often to prevent the spread of infection. The skin would crack and minor dermatitis was common from all the rough work and repeated washings. A patient who had active herpes could give it to the dentist's fingers, and then the dentist could spread it to other patients through hand-to-mouth contact. The *herpetic whitlow* (figure 11), or finger infection, was a well-established occupational hazard for dentists. The dentist unlucky enough to get herpes on the finger could, in turn, give it to patients by continuing to work without gloves. Dentists (and dental hygienists and dental assistants) now wear gloves at all times when working in the mouths of patients to avoid herpes and other infections. Gloves should also be worn by other health care professionals such as nurses and respiratory therapists, who often touch their patients' mouths.

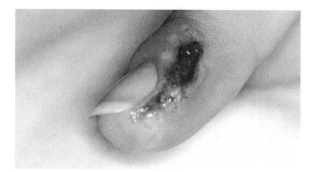

Figure 11: Herpetic whitlow. Finger infections with herpes can be caused by type 1 or type 2 virus. They may be severe or mild, frequent or infrequent. If tender areas recur on your hand, let your doctor know. These lesions will develop at the site of inoculation of the virus, and may appear on the finger tips, or in several other places on the hand as depicted in these photographs.

Who else can get a herpetic whitlow? Anyone whose ungloved hands touch the face or mouth or genitals of another person.

Thus, the list includes doctors, nurses, respiratory therapists, wrestlers, and rugby players. Herpes may become a problem in any contact sport. It has been known to affect many players on the same team. What happens to the players on a team just before a big challenging event? If you believe in emotional stress as a trigger for herpes, you will expect that the event will trigger recurrences of sores that could peak with virus during the match. These special circumstances have resulted in special names: *herpes gladiatorum* occurs because the infected lips of one wrestler are rubbed, scrubbed, pushed, and plastered into the chest, legs, abdomen and other body parts of the opponent. In a rugby match, herpes called *herpes rugbeiforum* or *scrum pox* may form around the ears and scalp of players who contact other players' lips in the scrum. Herpes goes where it is inoculated, so sports can put herpes sores in all sorts of unusual places.

If your occupation has you sitting at a desk, standing at a teller's window, or working in the fields, herpes is not an occupational hazard. If you work as a technician in a diagnostic virus lab or as a dental hygienist, the situation is different. Remember the cardinal rule: herpes does not fly through the air with the greatest of ease. You cannot catch herpes from people who sit nearby you or share your toilet seat. However, if you commonly have skin-to-skin contact with others, and if the contact includes possible areas of active herpes, then the possibility of transmission is real. Add a little heat, broken skin, and moisture, as in a wrestling match or a dentist's chair, and transmission is likely.

10
Non-Genital
Herpes Infections

So went Satan forth from the presence of the Lord,
and smote Job with sore boils from the sole of
his foot unto his crown.

−JOB 2:7

Herpes of the face, mouth, and lips

The lip is the most common location for a herpes simplex infection of any kind. There are probably three to five times as many people with cold sores of the lip as there are people with genital herpes. It is a very common thing to see a facial herpes outbreak. Look at people at the beach on the first day of bright sunshine or at skiers on the slopes on the first day of snow. The sun triggers the recurrence of fever blisters, most commonly on the vermilion border— the border between the skin of the face and the thinner, pinker mucus membrane of the lips and mouth (see figure 12, page 202).

The fever blister is the recurrent form of herpes of the face. It may erupt repeatedly. Facial sores behave similarly to genital sores. Recurrences range from frequent to nonexistent and usually decrease in frequency with time. Facial sores have active phases with warnings (prodromes) followed by sores. Because the skin around the lips is a bit drier than the skin of the genitals, the vesicle (blister) stage is more common.

The classical tale of transmission of oral-facial herpes is as follows: an adult relative transmits herpes to a child by kissing or by sharing an article such as a drinking glass. Facial infection could come from any oral-to-oral contact during childhood or adulthood. Herpes simplex virus does not care where it is inoculated, just as long as it gets inoculated. Thus, oral herpes resulting from genital-to-oral contact is becoming more common.

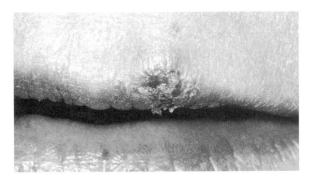

Figure 12: A recurrence of oral herpes simplex (herpes labialis). Oral or facial herpes is commonly found at the tip of the nostrils and around the nose or elsewhere on the face. Instead of recurring by reactivation of herpes simplex from the sacral ganglion, facial herpes recurs from reactivation of virus latent in the trigeminal ganglion.

Like primary herpes infection anywhere, primary facial herpes is usually more severe than recurrent facial herpes. The skin sores are more numerous and more painful. Sores at the back of the throat can cause a sore throat. Severe primary mouth infection in a child commonly results in gingivostomatitis, in which almost the whole mouth becomes a target for the virus. Ulcers burst out everywhere in the mouth and may make swallowing food very difficult. Lymph nodes (glands) in the neck may also be swollen and tender. For the usual primary period of two to three weeks, the person is miserable. It may be necessary to use topical anesthetics like lidocaine (Xylocaine) to help swallowing. Children who suck their thumbs need to stop this habit immediately if they have this infection, in order to avoid painful autoinoculation to the fingers (herpetic whitlow).

Just as with herpes on other parts of the body, oral herpes infections are usually not noticed by the person who has them. In such asymptomatic cases, the primary or first infection on the face passes unnoticed or is thought to be some other illness. If the child has gingivostomatitis, generally it will be easily diagnosed. If the child has only a sore throat or a little fever, the whole event may pass unnoticed until the first recurrence. Then the cold sore or fever blister raises its little vesicles on the face. The virus usually reactivates near the lip, but the nose, the cheeks, and even the earlobe are fair game. The rules for oral herpes are like those for genital herpes:

1. Oral herpes is active during active phases. During those phases avoid kissing, especially newborn babies. Also avoid oral sex, thumb sucking, nose picking, and eye rubbing.

2. Keep contact lenses out of your mouth at all times, especially when cold sores are active.

3. Stay away from your dentist when you have a cold sore. It would not be nice for the dentist.

4. What about treatment? Many of the same rules apply here as for genital herpes, so they will not be repeated. Effective treatment for an active cold sore is now possible. Topical penciclovir (Denavir, Vectravir) will reduce the pain and shorten the time required for healing to occur. Oral acyclovir suppression (continuous treatment) is beneficial for people with frequent recurrences or during periods of exposure to known trigger factors (especially sun exposure). Aside from topical penciclovir and suppression with oral acyclovir, no other effective treatments have yet been identified. Many possible treatments are undergoing research trials. Prescription medicines such as acyclovir ointment (the U.S. formulation) and idoxuridine drops are not effective. A cream formulation of acyclovir is sold in Europe and Canada for cold sores and may be better than the ointment for this purpose, but more studies are needed. The whole matter is very confusing when you go to the drugstore because there are at least a dozen "cold sore" products that claim to "speed healing" or provide "relief." These products do not use the word "herpes" in their claims because they have no proven benefit against this virus. While unlikely to cause harm, most "cold sore" products on the drugstore shelves are ineffective.

5. To soothe the affected area, use a warm, wet face cloth to soak the area and then blow it dry with a hair dryer set on low. Do not use ice, ether, alcohol, BHT, soap, or petrolatum treatments.

Herpes of the eye

The course of infection of herpes of the eye is very much like the course of infection of herpes elsewhere. There is often a primary first episode with pain and swelling. Primary infections may be followed by recurrences. As with all herpes infections, recurrences cause less systemic (total body) involvement, and less tissue is upset, etc. However, recurrences in the eye may lead to local complications, which can interfere with vision. If the local complications become severe, decreased vision in the infected eye can result.

Generally, herpes of the eye is caused by herpes simplex type 1. The time of infection and source of virus are the same as with oral herpes. A baby or young child, more often than an adult, becomes infected with herpes simplex, generally through mouth contact— for example, a kiss from mom or dad. The person doing the kissing may have a fever blister or may not have a recognizable sore. When a small child falls and scrapes his or her face or forehead near the eye, and the child's mother kisses the scrape to make it better, herpes from the mother's mouth has ready-made access to epithelial cells in the cut. As far as the virus is concerned, this is as easy as using a needle for access; there are no barriers to jump across. Direct inoculation to the eye is also easy, because the barrier is generally so thin. The protective layer of the eye is not tough and thick like skin but rather thin and fragile. Transmission from genital sores on one person to the eye of another through direct contact of genitals to eye is possible though not common.

Primary herpes of the eye

Once herpes is inoculated, an infection may occur some two to twenty-one days later. The primary, or first, event with ocular (eye) herpes is characteristic yet sometimes difficult to diagnose. Generally (though not always), only one eye is affected. Redness and discomfort of the eye develops. This is the appearance of pinkeye or *conjunctivitis*. The sac protecting the eye is inflamed. When you pull down the bag under your eye and look into the mirror, you are looking at the membrane called the conjunctiva. Conjunctivitis is an extremely common infection in children. In most cases, the virus causing it is not herpes simplex. A very common cause of conjunctivitis in children is *adenovirus*, which commonly occurs in small epidemics or outbreaks at swimming pools, schools, and so forth. Unlike herpes simplex, adenovirus is a very hardy virus, capable of withstanding drying; it flies through the air with the greatest of ease. Adenovirus usually involves both eyes. Other viruses, bacteria, and Chlamydia can also cause conjunctivitis. In the case of herpes, along with the redness and discomfort comes a watery discharge. Often the neck glands are swollen and a lymph node just to the front of the ear on the same side as the eye infection is inflamed and tender. The eyelid of the infected eye may be swollen. Often (though not always) a careful search for typical herpes lesions (see pictures referred to in chapter 3) will yield a positive result. Herpes lesions are sometimes found on the eyelid, under the eyelashes, on the forehead, in the hair, near the nose, or near the mouth.

At this point, the person may feel sick, but vision is normal. The whole process of conjunctivitis lasts about two or three weeks. An ophthalmologist (eye specialist) may choose to prescribe antiviral (antiherpes) eye drops. There is no information proving that treatment at this point is effective or even helpful in preventing more severe eye involvement. Despite that, if it were my eye, I'd put in the drops.

Usually herpes conjunctivitis just heals at that stage and that's it. Primary herpes occasionally affects the cornea, however. If this happens, the symptoms described for conjunctivitis are just beginning to clear when new, quite different, symptoms begin. During herpes conjunctivitis, vision is not affected. As *keratitis* (inflammation of the cornea) begins, however, vision may blur. Blurred vision resulting from herpes means the cornea is inflamed. The cornea is a protective outer coat of transparent material that covers the front of the eye where light enters. It is the part just under a contact lens. Keratitis, which may also begin with no history of conjunctivitis, is a much more serious problem than conjunctivitis,

THE TRUTH ABOUT HERPES

because we look through the cornea (see figure 13), whereas the conjunctiva is a protective membrane that we don't actually look through. Inflammation of the cornea leads to blurred vision. If a deep opaque scar of the cornea were to develop, decreased vision in the eye might result. Universally, with keratitis, the eye feels gritty to its owner, as if it had a sandpaper surface, and it responds to bright light with a spasm of pain called *photophobia*.

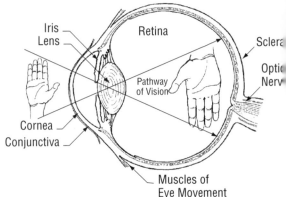

Figure 13: The anatomy of the eye. The conjunctiva, which forms a protective outer sac around the front of the eye (sort of like "eye skin"), is the first place for herpes of the eye to affect. Recurrences can be a problem because of involvement of the cornea, since the cornea is part of the visual pathway. If the cornea is blurred, the vision may be blurred. If only the conjunctiva is affected, vision is not blurred.

Iris
Lens
Retina
Sclera
Optic Nerv
Pathway of Vision
Cornea
Conjunctiva
Muscles of Eye Movement

If you suspect keratitis, go to an ophthalmologist. The tests for the diagnosis of keratitis can only be done properly by someone with the right equipment and experience in eye diseases. In order to see the lesion properly, the specialist uses a slit lamp, which is a sort of rotating microscope, to see an enlarged view of your eye as you hold your head still on a resting post. A dye called rose bengal or fluorescein will be used to make a herpes sore stand out clearly. The diagnosis of herpes depends mostly on the specialist's opinion, although he or she may do a virus test.

If herpes simplex is confirmed, it can be treated with several things:

1. An antiviral agent. Several good antiherpes drugs can be used in the eye. Locally applied drugs help a lot in the eye, often a very different situation from herpes elsewhere. Useful drugs for the eye include idoxuridine (IDU, Stoxil, Herplex), adenine arabinoside (ara-A, Vira-A), and trifluorothymidine (TFT, Viroptic, Trifluridine). Systemic (intravenous or oral) acyclovir

is also being used more frequently in this setting. A host of other chemicals are being developed for use here. It is arguable which drug should be used first and why. A specialist physician should be consulted in case of herpes of the eye, and his or her advice should be carefully followed.

2. A cycloplegic. This drug relaxes a muscle in the eye called the ciliary muscle and causes the eye to dilate and relax just as it does when you get drops at the eye doctor's office. It reduces photophobia.

3. Various pain relievers are useful here.

4. Sunglasses or very dark glasses may help.

5. Early keratitis is often treated with *debridement*, a minor surgical cleaning procedure that is quite helpful for early keratitis. It is not used in later stages of keratitis.

Recurrent herpes of the eye

Primary herpes of the eye generally causes only two or three weeks of conjunctivitis and does not affect vision. As the conjunctivitis improves, some people get keratitis, which can cause further problems. When ocular herpes recurs, it does so by causing recurrent keratitis. Eventually, the feeling of grittiness and pain may decrease, because herpes of the eye causes a loss of feeling of the eye surface (cornea) called *hypoesthesia*. Instead there may be a recurrence of irritation, as though something like sand or dust is in the eye. With each recurrence there may be an increase in tearing. There may be a recurrence of photophobia. Sores may also appear on the lips, face, mouth, or nose. The eye specialist will assess each recurrence to make sure it is herpes.

You may be treated with the same drugs listed for primary herpes of the eye. Drops of cortisone or any of its derivatives, which are absolutely contraindicated during conjunctivitis and early keratitis, may be useful when carefully administered during some deeper forms of keratitis called *disciform keratitis* or *stromal keratitis*. (An incomplete list of cortisone drops includes Betnesol, Cortisporin, Decadron, Mitered, Metreton, Neo-Cortef, Neo-Medrol,

Optimyd, and Sofracort.) Generally, cortisone drops are combined with a specific antiviral drug so that the virus growth is held back. The eye specialist may wish to repeatedly perform debridement. Oral acyclovir is increasingly used in the systemic treatment and/or prevention of herpes keratitis. In preliminary studies, it appears to be very effective and might be considered for anyone whose herpes keratitis is frequent or causing a lot of cosmetic or sight problems. It is generally used, in selected cases, as a continuous suppressive treatment. Oral acyclovir does not replace the other eye treatments listed above. There has not been enough experience yet with the new agents to make a specific recommendation.

Herpes encephalitis

Encephalitis means inflammation of the brain tissue. It is different from *meningitis*, which means inflammation of the *meninges*—the protective sac around the brain. In *meningoencephalitis*, both brain tissue and meninges become infected at the same time with the same agent. Herpes simplex can cause either encephalitis or meningitis. The outcomes are very different.

Herpes encephalitis in an adult is a very serious disease. Without treatment, encephalitis is often deadly. With treatment, it may also be deadly or may cause significant brain damage. It does not have any correlation whatsoever to herpes of the mucus membrane, skin, or eyes. It is a disease of its own that occurs for reasons we do not understand. People with genital herpes are neither prone to nor protected from herpes encephalitis.

Herpes meningitis should not be confused with encephalitis. Meningitis is a direct complication of genital or anal herpes. It commonly occurs as a symptom of primary herpes and may cause severe headache or photophobia. It does not cause permanent damage to the nervous system. Left alone, herpes meningitis gets better and almost never recurs. Treated, it also gets better and almost never recurs.

Herpes encephalitis may also occur during neonatal herpes. The symptoms and prevention of neonatal herpes are discussed in chapter 6. Neonatal herpes encephalitis usually, though not always, follows genital herpes in the mother. Most mothers who give birth to babies with this problem did not know they had herpes. It is important to identify pregnant women who have genital herpes, especially those whose genital herpes is primary, because studies show that neonatal herpes can be prevented quite effectively by cesarean section if herpes is active.

Herpes encephalitis of the adult occurs by an altogether different mechanism. Science has not been able to fully explain how herpes simplex makes its way to the brain. It may get there by a number of ways, most likely by traveling up the olfactory nerve, which runs above the nose, inside the skull, and at the base of the front of the brain. Normally, herpes of the face, lip, nose, or eye travels along the trigeminal nerve and then stops at the trigeminal ganglion, where it stays as a latent infection (see chapter 2). In encephalitis, however, the virus usually reactivates from its latency stop somewhere in the olfactory-temporal pathway of the brain. From there, it travels or reactivates right in the brain tissue itself—usually in the temporal lobe, more or less underneath the temple or the ear. Herpes encephalitis is rare and is seen both in people who have facial herpes and in people who do not. The virus stays in the temporal lobe and directly damages just the area of the lobe it is in. In doing so, however, it causes swelling and inflammation that can result in more widespread damage. Because the brain is enclosed in a hard casing of bone with no extra room, any swelling that occurs inside the skull causes the brain to be compressed. Because the temporal lobe controls emotions and other important functions, damage to this area can cause a series of problems. A change in consciousness ranging from sleepiness or disorientation to deep coma is nearly universal. Early in the course of infection, there may be headache. Commonly, there is a sudden personality change or bizarre behavior. A seizure (fit, convulsion) may occur. Speech may be abnormal. Paralysis or weakness on one side of the body sometimes occurs. In most cases, paralysis like this results not from herpes but from stroke.

Herpes encephalitis occurs at any age from infancy to old age. In adults and older children, there is fever in 90 percent of cases. Herpes encephalitis is often extremely difficult to diagnose. Several tests may be performed in the search for the answer, among them electroencephalography (EEG), computerized tomography (CT scan), and a brain scan. Unfortunately, none of these tests is specific.

As with all herpes infections, the diagnosis depends on finding the virus. In the case of herpes encephalitis, the herpes simplex virus is in brain tissue only. New technology allows earlier diagnosis of this disease. A specialized DNA technique called the *polymerase chain reaction*, or PCR, is so sensitive that it can find the trace of just a few viral molecules of DNA in a sample by amplifying the signal through a chain reaction method. This technique is now moving from research laboratories into clinical laboratories as it becomes more useful to clinicians for diagnosis of many infections. However, because of the sensitivity of PCR, scientists have been plagued by positives that occur even when the virus is not active. We do not yet fully understand the value of PCR tests in genital herpes. Viral culture, which is already the gold standard of diagnosis, shows a positive result and then shows a negative result in accordance with the disappearance of symptoms. Early reports from laboratories performing the PCR test on genital skin show that this test is frequently positive when the viral culture is negative. Some components of the virus are present on the skin at times when virus cannot be grown in the laboratory. The significance of this is yet to be determined. Sometimes a very sensitive test is precisely what is required. For example, it is never expected to find any evidence of herpes by any test—no matter how sensitive—in a protected area of the body like the spinal fluid. Therefore, finding a positive PCR test in that area usually means that a clinical disease is present. A positive PCR from the mouth or genital area, however, does not necessarily mean that *active* disease is present. The test only confirms that the person has herpes affecting that area, not whether the virus is currently active, culturable, or transmissible. It shows merely that the DNA fingerprint has been identified in the area. PCR test results are an added piece of evidence which must be interpreted within the context of the whole clinical situation. PCR is now the best way of making an early diagnosis of encephalitis.

The treatment for herpes encephalitis is intravenous acyclovir (Zovirax), which is quite helpful in decreasing a death rate that is otherwise 75 percent in biopsy-proven cases. It is not a miraculous therapy for everyone, because damage may have been done to vital brain tissue before therapy has had the chance to work. Now that the PCR test is making this diagnosis easier, without biopsy, herpes encephalitis is a much less frightening and serious disease. Herpes encephalitis is very uncommon in adults and has absolutely no connection to genital herpes.

11
Therapy
Now and Later

For every evil under the sun
There is a remedy or there is none
If there be one, seek till you find it
If there be none, never mind it.

—MOTHER GOOSE

There's never been a better time to have genital herpes. Several safe treatments are now available that have proven themselves through clinical trials and clinical practice to be hightly effective at treating herpes outbreaks, preventing recurrences, and preventing asymptomatic shedding.

You may want to share this chapter with your doctor. Much of it may seem rather technical. Knowing about the molecular mechanisms of antiherpes drugs and the results of recent clinical trials is not essential to understanding your herpes.

Accepted therapy today: What can I do right now?

If you have a first episode of genital herpes or think you may have:

1. Go to your doctor or clinic as soon as possible. Early diagnosis and treatment will help you to feel substantially better more quickly.

2. Have a trained professional diagnose the problem and confirm the presence of herpes by a virus test taken from the affected area (a culture test with typing is preferred, but a direct antigen test or an electron microscope test is also acceptable).

3. A blood test for syphilis, HIV, and possibly hepatitis B should

212

also be performed. The syphilis test should be repeated in a couple of weeks and the HIV and hepatitis B tests repeated in several months.

4. If the pain is severe, you may wish to take a prescription pain reliever.

5. Take very warm showers to run warm water over the area three or four times a day. Occasionally people find water on these sores to be absolutely intolerable. If that happens to you, stop using water. Most people find water very helpful, however.

6. When you get out of the shower or bath, blow the genital area dry with a hair dryer. Set the temperature on low or cool, and be careful not to burn yourself.

7. Make sure you are passing urine without difficulty. If you try and it won't come, try again. Try urinating in the shower or tub to decrease the sting. Turn on the sink tap for background noise. Outside the bath, you might try to direct the urine stream away from your sores with a bit of rolled up toilet tissue. Pouring a glass of warm water over the area may also be helpful. Some people have found that drinking a lot of water (eight glasses a day) dilutes the urine enough that it hurts less. Others point out that this increases the number of times you have to urinate. Whether you would rather it hurt more intensely on fewer occasions or less intensely on more occasions is up to you.

8. If you cannot pass urine and you've tried several times, wait a couple of hours—even three or four. If there is still no result, you must have medical attention. Not passing urine can lead to serious problems, which are totally preventable. Either visit your own doctor or go to the emergency room of a local hospital.

9. Avoid wearing tight underwear. If possible, do without underwear altogether. Try wearing loose clothes made of pure cotton. When you get home, take a shower or soak in the tub. Leave your clothes off if you can.

10. You should be treated by your physician with acyclovir (Zovirax) or one of the new antiviral agents that have also been

proven to be effective for the treatment of primary genital herpes. One is valacyclovir (Valtrex; 500 to 1,000 mg twice daily) and the other is famciclovir (Famvir; 250 mg three times daily). They are discussed later in this chapter. Generally, one of these three drugs should be taken orally as soon as the diagnosis of a first episode of genital herpes is suspected. Treatment is usually continued for seven to ten days or for longer if the lesions are not healed by then. In some countries, it is customary to treat first episodes for as few as five to seven days. Continuing to take one of these medicines after five to seven days is much less important than starting it as soon as possible during a first clinical episode. A topical (ointment) preparation of acyclovir is also available but is much less effective than the oral form and should not be used for first episodes. If you are having your first clinical episode of herpes, the topical preparations currently available are not effective enough. If hospitalization is necessary, acyclovir can be given intravenously, although this is rarely necessary. If your outbreak is quite severe and is giving you trouble walking, or if your head feels like the top is going to come off, or if you are having trouble urinating, then hospitalization may be required. More information on acyclovir and other new antiviral drugs is given later in this chapter.

11. Avoid (because they may be worse than doing nothing):
    • cortisone cream or ointment
    • antibiotic cream or ointment
    • any cream or ointment that does not contain a useful, specific antiherpes drug
    • petrolatum (e.g., Vaseline)
    • antibiotics (unless you have a clear-cut secondary infection)
    • alcohol (because it stings)
    • ether (because it stings and can catch fire)
    • DMSO (dimethyl sulfoxide)

    Avoid (because they are of no proven benefit):
    • L-lysine
    • BHT
    • idoxuridine (IDU, Stoxil, Herplex-D)

12. If you have first episode herpes during pregnancy, tell your physician and read chapter 6 of this book. Take care of yourself by giving yourself time to heal, treating any other infections, and treating your herpes. Even though you are pregnant, discuss the possibility of taking acyclovir if you are having a true primary episode.

13. It is hard to learn and figure out everything all at once, but the answers will come. Your ability to cope and your methods for coping will also evolve. There is no truth to the rumor that stress will make your primary herpes worse. It is very distressing to have primary herpes. Accept the stress for now. Follow the suggestions above to take care of the immediate problem.

After my first episode herpes is over

At this point, it is usually not clear what your pattern of recurrences will be. Generally, most people with type 2 herpes will get recurrences. Type 1 also recurs, although generally much less frequently than type 2. Latent infection inside the ganglion does not hurt you, and it is not curable by any drug, at present. For now, it is not possible to intervene and control latent infection with a drug.

What if I am having recurrent herpes?

People with recurrent genital herpes now have choices to make regarding antiviral treatment for control of the infection. To make informed choices, it is necessary to understand about how treatments are studied to determine if they are safe and effective. As a consumer of drug treatments or nutritional supplements—whether by prescription or over the counter—it is good to understand what it is you are buying. During the first episode, it is almost always a good idea to use systemic antiviral treatment if it is available to you. This treatment lasts only a short time and is very effective. After the first episode infection is over, however, the effects of treatment depend on three key factors:

1. The nature (frequency, severity) of your herpes recurrences.

2. The proven effectiveness of the treatment in controlled clinical trials.

3. Using the treatment for what it is intended to do.

With recurrent herpes, it is important to fully understand the active phases of infection so you can avoid sore-to-skin contact when necessary (see chapter 3). It is also important to use safer sex precautions for the prevention of herpes and all other sexually transmitted diseases (see chapter 12). If you are facing issues such as loneliness and the fear of discussing herpes with new partners, keep in mind that these are very common issues and that frustrations can be overcome through a commitment to yourself and to your ability to grow from this experience. In addition, you may wish to have treatment for recurrent herpes. Before you decide that you do or don't want treatment, read the rest of this chapter, on various aspects of treatment. You should be sure that you are clear about your objectives in deciding to use or avoid medication. Some people who would benefit immensely from safe and effective therapy avoid it for the wrong reasons; others take medication in the wrong way and receive minimal benefits. I have seen many people give up on a very effective treatment because they become frustrated when it does not work, and it turns out that it does not work because they are taking the treatment incorrectly. Several advances have been made in the past ten years in the medical management of genital herpes. If treatment can benefit you, why not give it a try? On the other hand, if you find that treatment would not do much for you, why bother?

What is a clinical trial and what are the goals of treatment?

A clinical trial is a test of a new treatment done under special experimental conditions on consenting human subjects. Today, in studying genital herpes, a new drug is considered effective only if it can satisfy some basic requirements:

1. It must be safe and effective at killing virus *in vitro*—in the test tube—or else safe and effective in animals experimentally infected with herpes. Drugs that are not intended to kill the herpes virus but rather to boost the body's natural immunity would be ineffective in the test tube but would have to show an effect in the animal model.

2. It must be studied for use in herpes in a double-blind, placebo-controlled, randomized trial. The trial is called double-blind because both the volunteers and the investigator are blind as to which volunteer is getting which therapy; that is, neither knows which volunteers are getting the real drug and which are getting a placebo (a treatment look-alike without the medicine) until the end of the trial. The placebo control drug looks like, tastes like, and smells like the real drug. The study is randomized by a statistician, so that there is no possible way to predict which volunteers receive the real drug.

Indications of whether the drug is useful—for example, the appearance of sores, the duration of sores, the pain and itching of sores, and the duration of virus in sores—are monitored very closely.

Certain factors known to affect the course of the illness are grouped together for study. For example, since recurrent herpes lasts about one week and primary herpes about three, it is clear that primary and recurrent herpes must not be compared to each other; rather, they must be separately studied.

Results of the drug testing are tabulated and then locked into a computer. Once the results are locked in, the code is broken. Then the statisticians, scientists, and physicians can analyze whether the people who got the drug responded in a different way from the group who got the placebo. If the drug works better than the placebo, conclusions can be drawn about whether the drug will be useful or not. If the effect is "statistically significant"—mathematically clear—the effect of the drug is unlikely to have occurred as a result of chance alone.

The average recurrence of genital herpes lasts only about five or six days from start to finish. The time from start to finish is so short that it is very difficult to construct clinical trials that can measure changes caused by treatments. If we measure the natural duration of viral shedding from a skin sore in a recurrent episode without using any treatment at all, we find that about half of all people stop shedding virus on their own about forty-eight hours after their episode has started. Until 1992, there had never been a published study of a treatment for genital herpes even checked for changes in patients more than every twenty-four hours, and even that frequency was considered very high.

So even the best clinical trials of drugs for treatment of recurrent genital herpes need to be interpreted with a grain of salt, since the observation points have often been too far apart to detect benefits. In a recurrent episode, what must a drug accomplish if it is going to be considered a success and warrant general use? The ideal drug would have virtually no toxicity or bad side effects, would work immediately at the time of the first dose, could be taken during the warning phase of a herpes episode, and would prevent the episode entirely. Recently, a Canadian study of famciclovir (Famvir) showed that early treatment before the start of viral shedding (during the prodrome) significantly reduced the number of people who shed virus for that episode. A study of valacyclovir showed that it could increase the proportion of people who do not develop the vesicle-ulcer stage of herpes.

In considering aborted episodes (defined a bit differently in each study) as a drug effect, we have to be especially careful, since studies without treatment have shown that one or two of every five episodes are aborted naturally. It is crucial that people consider not only the effect they observe in themselves but also the scientific results and findings. It is very easy to believe that you are using a strong medicine when, in fact, it is just that your body's immune system fights off recurrent herpes quite well on its own. Both famciclovir and valacyclovir have shown effects that stand up to scientific trial standards. However, neither drug should be expected to abort most episodes.

An antiviral medication designed to kill herpes simplex virus on the spot should be able to demonstrate its antiviral abilities in comparison to a placebo in a clinical trial, and it should be able to lessen the normal duration and severity of an untreated episode. Even if a drug shows a good antiviral effect, it can be very difficult to demonstrate that the drug makes episodes shorter and/or less severe. Scientists are currently not sure why this is so. Part of the reason is the great variability between people and between episodes in the same person. An episode that hurts a lot and lasts for ten days can be followed by another episode that only tingles a bit and lasts for three days.

One of the biggest problems with herpes clinical trials is that 20 to 30 percent of episodes that occur are actually culture-negative, even though they occur in a person known to have proven recurrent genital herpes. Culture-negative sores may appear to be herpes even to an experienced investigator, but virus is not grown from the sores. To date, all clinical trials for recurrent herpes have included culture-negative sores in their analyses. We do not know why culture-negative episodes occur, but we know that they are much shorter and less severe than the same person's culture-positive episodes. The question is how an antiviral medication can be expected to have an effect on an episode that lacks virus.

Another example of practical problems arising in clinical trials results from the fact that men and women differ a lot in the way their sores appear. Men generally experience lesions on dry skin. They also tend to experience and complain of pain quite differently than women. One way of getting around these is to look for "swab tenderness." This measures how much a herpes sore hurts when you poke at it with a cotton swab. Women tend to skip the vesicle phase because their sores tend to come up on skin that is somewhat wet, making it very difficult for the vesicles to form. Another pitfall in study design occurs when a new drug is applied too late in the course of an outbreak. Under such circumstances, a drug benefit is very unlikely to be identified because the window of opportunity for early treatment has been missed.

In general, the clinical investigator must take every possible effort to reduce the expected level of variability through careful study design in order to be certain that the observed effects of a new drug are an accurate reflection of the truth. Conversely, a study that fails to find a drug benefit that is present is also not helping the patient who needs treatment.

I only get recurrences every three or four months. Is there a cream or salve I can use instead of oral medication?

Topical acyclovir (Zovirax) ointment has been extensively studied in the treatment of recurrent herpes, but unfortunately it is not well absorbed through the skin and has not been shown to be effective enough for recurrent herpes to justify its use for that purpose in the majority of patients. Nevertheless, I have seen several patients who swear that topical acyclovir is helpful. This could be because there is some variability in its effectiveness; it works for some people and not for others. However, it could also be that people who believe in this treatment are not truly receiving a benefit that could be demonstrated. In some studies, topical acyclovir ointment did kill the herpes virus a little more quickly during recurrences than a placebo. Concerning topical acyclovir, however, Dr. Richard Reichman and his coworkers reported in the *Journal of Infectious Diseases* the following results of a carefully conducted trial: "There were no significant differences between the [topical] acyclovir and placebo-treated groups of either sex in time to crusting of lesions, time required for lesions to heal, time to cessation of pain, or in the frequency with which new lesions developed during their course of therapy. Mild, transient burning or pain associated with application of the study medication was a common complaint." In actually getting rid of lesions, topical acyclovir is not generally useful. Additional studies have demonstrated that using topical acyclovir even very early, starting it at the first warning sign of recurrence (prodrome), has no useful clinical effect. In certain parts of the world, acyclovir is available as a water-soluble cream rather than an ointment. One study suggested a therapeutic benefit for the cream preparation. In fact, there is slightly better drug absorption when it is used this way, so a greater effect might be expected. Unfortunately, there are very few well-controlled clinical trials to report on the aqueous cream. It is not yet available in the United States, but is marketed in Canada and Europe. If you have tried it topically and it is not working for you, you should not feel that the drug, itself, is ineffective. Perhaps your recurrence pattern would be more effectively treated with the same drug given in a different way. Acyclovir is much more effective when it is taken by mouth (tablets, capsules, or syrup), depending on various factors, as outlined later in this chapter.

There is a current role for topical treatment of recurrent genital herpes, however. In the future, topical treatments hold even more promise. Two different antivirals used topically have been shown to have some beneficial effects in recurrent herpes. These two agents are high dose *alpha interferon* and 3 percent *edoxudine cream* (Virostat). Neither agent is a major breakthrough. Both have shown enough benefit in clinical trial to warrant use, in my opinion, by people who choose to try a topical agent for short-term relief of discomfort during recurrences. They are beneficial and not harmful. Should a person spend money on a treatment that is beneficial but does not exactly offer cure? This is something that only the individual person can answer. I can see several reasons why an effective topical agent for recurrent herpes would offer a lot of people an answer they seek. First, currently available oral therapy is most effective for first episodes and frequent recurrences. Second, many people would prefer to use a topical agent, if given the choice, rather than an oral agent, since the topical agent stays at the site of the infection. Third, application of a soothing agent that is also helpful in healing could be a nice thing to do to help one feel better sooner. Personally, I feel that we have neglected a very important area by not pursuing topical treatment more aggressively. Further advances in this field are expected in the next five years or so, however, and I am sure that eventually topical treatment will be a major treatment used by many people.

Two studies have demonstrated some clinical benefits with topical alpha interferon, which is a naturally occurring antiviral agent made by immune cells in the human body. Its effects are slightly delayed because it must induce secondary agents from the body's own defense system to be effective. Nevertheless, studies using slightly different preparations have demonstrated a significant antiviral effect. One study used a "recombinant" preparation of interferon using a human gene growing in yeast cells and made by large-scale fermentation, while the other used a preparation of interferon made directly from the white blood cells of human blood donors. The two studies showed about the same findings. First, benefits from topical interferon are definitely dose-dependent, and the dose has to be fairly high to be effective. Second, there is no apparent harm in using the high dose. Both preparations, at high dose, have significant antiviral effects and reduce certain symptoms. Neither preparation was actually able to demonstrate a shortening of recurrences' duration. This could be partly attributed to the interferon itself, which is known to delay healing a bit.

Edoxudine is a nucleoside antiviral agent that works similarly to acyclovir, except that it loses its effectiveness when given systemically, because an enzyme in the body (pyrimidine nucleoside phosphorylase) acts directly upon this drug to immediately break it apart. This action could actually be an advantage for a topical agent, since the drug is not absorbed intact, theoretically reducing any risk from a circulating intact drug. Edoxudine is a bit less effective *in vitro* (in a test tube) compared with acyclovir. However, the topical preparation may get to its target more effectively. Edoxudine cream at a concentration of 3 percent is effective at treating herpes infections in non-human animal models and has been shown to be effective at significantly reducing the duration of viral shedding in studies of people with genital herpes. Edoxudine cream studies also showed some other benefits to human volunteers with genital herpes, specifically a reduction in the duration of lesion tenderness. This effect was seen best in women; the authors concluded in the *Journal of Infectious Diseases* in 1991 that five days' treatment with topical edoxudine 3 percent cream reduced viral shedding in men by about one day and in women by about one and one-half days. Loss of observed signs was improved by nearly two days and lesion discomfort was also shortened somewhat in edoxudine-treated women. Edoxudine was well tolerated and reduced several signs of herpes in women. Its clinical role in recurrent genital herpes remains to be fully determined. It is currently in use in some parts of Europe under a different brand name (Aedurid) and is available in Canada by prescription. Eventually, these preparations may be available in other countries. The benefits of treatment remain moderate, however, and so whether or not to use it is still an individual choice. Topical edoxudine is not a replacement for chronic suppression of frequent recurrences or a replacement for oral or intravenous treatment for primary episodes. Although autoinoculation is unlikely to occur during a recurrence, you would be wise to use a swab, a glove, or a finger cot whenever you use a topical agent for herpes that is in an active phase of infection. If you have herpes only occasionally you can now choose from several oral treatments that offer clinical benefits when taken early in an episode. You also have the option of taking medication on a continuous basis (suppression).

Although some benefits have been seen with creams and ointments, the benefits of certain oral medications (discussed in the next section) are more predictable. Although direct comparisons between topicals and tablets have not been made, it is currently a better choice to opt for one of the oral antiviral agents until more powerful topical treatments become available.

The oral antiviral treatments: How do they work?

Acyclovir:

In December 1977, Gertrude Elion, a biochemist, and Howard Schaeffer, a chemist, along with four coworkers, announced their discovery of a new chemical compound. These scientists from Wellcome Research Laboratories called it by its chemical name 9-(2-hydroxyethoxymethyl) guanine. It was also known by the code name BW248U and the descriptive name acycloguanosine, which was modified to the official generic term acyclovir. The compound now carries the trade name Zovirax. Dr. Schaeffer and Ms. Elion won the 1988 Nobel Prize in Physiology and Medicine for their discovery of acyclovir as well as for discoveries of several other very important drugs for controlling infectious, malignant, and metabolic disease.

In 1985, acyclovir was released in oral form for use by people with genital herpes infections, marking the beginning of a new era of therapy for genital herpes. Until then, home remedies had been the rule. Dietary supplements, food additives, and a host of other treatments were used (most often unsuccessfully) to try to change the frequency of recurrences. The story is different now. It has been proven beyond any doubt that oral acyclovir does the following:

1. Taken for five days, beginning at the outset of a recurrence of genital herpes, acyclovir shortens the episode.

2. Taken every day, in doses ranging from two to five capsules or tablets per day, acyclovir prevents most outbreaks and reduces the severity of the episodes that break through. The most common dosage is 400 mg twice daily.

3. Taken during the first episode of genital herpes, acyclovir shortens the episode by one week on average and lessens the severity of urinary discomfort and swollen lymph nodes.

These dramatic clinical findings make a big difference to many people who have problems with their herpes infections. For those who need it, oral acyclovir can be a very effective treatment.

Now two new drugs are available to treat and/or suppress herpes infections. This section outlines how these drugs work and how they affect the virus and the human body—the information you'll need to know when deciding with your physician whether you want to try one of them. The doses and indications for use are not necessarily those described in the official drug inserts. As always, it is with your own physician that you must decide on the course of action you will take, after all of the particulars of your specific situation have been taken into account.

Famciclovir and valacyclovir (see plate 16, page 102):

Famciclovir (Famvir) is a new oral antiviral agent made by SmithKline Beecham Pharma. When ingested, most if not all of the famciclovir is converted quickly in the intestine and the liver to the active drug penciclovir. Therefore, famciclovir is called the *prodrug* of penciclovir. Famciclovir is used because it is very highly absorbed by the mouth: about 77 percent of this prodrug is absorbed compared with only about 15 percent of acyclovir. Because of the excellent oral absorption of famciclovir, penciclovir gets to the site of infection more quickly and to a greater extent than orally administered penciclovir or acyclovir. Famciclovir has been studied in first episodes and recurrent episodes. Its effects are outlined in the following sections.

Penciclovir is under study as an intravenous preparation, but it is not yet available for that use. Topical penciclovir is also effective at reducing sores and symptoms in a 1 percent cream formulation as a treatment for herpes labialis or cold sores.

Valacyclovir is a new oral formulation of acyclovir manufactured by Glaxo Wellcome, Inc. Like famciclovir, valacyclovir is well-absorbed—55 percent is absorbed. Upon absorption, this drug is almost completely converted in the liver to acyclovir by an enzyme called valacyclovir hydrolase. The mechanism of action and the potential effects and side effects of valacyclovir are therefore identical to acyclovir with the exception that acyclovir is available at the site of infection more quickly and to a much greater extent than if it were administered orally. The amount of acyclovir that gets into the body is three to four times the amount after oral acyclovir tablets are swallowed. The intravenous form of valacyclovir is still the old standard, acyclovir.

Mechanisms of action:
These drugs all work at the site of infection by mimicking a molecule called deoxyguanosine, one of the building blocks of DNA. Chemically, deoxyguanosine is a member of the class of compounds known as *nucleosides*, so these drugs are all known as nucleoside analogs. In many ways, they behave just like deoxyguanosine. Four nucleosides in all are used by the cells in our bodies to make DNA. DNA (which, because of its shape, is also called the double helix) is the hereditary material—the code transmitted from parent to child—that determines many characteristics, from the shape of your nose to the color of your skin. Every cell in every part of the human body contains DNA. In many of these cells, DNA rapidly divides in order to create new cells from old. Even though we may have stopped growing in overall size, many of our cells, such as sperm cells and white blood cells that fight off infection, need constant replacing. Stomach and intestinal cells are also continuously sloughed off as dead and then digested and replaced with new cells containing new DNA. Our bodies are constantly being replaced and reproduced in small cellular bits. These cellular reproductive processes all require healthy, intact DNA as the basic code for the continuation of the system.

The herpes simplex virus also uses double-stranded DNA as its basic coding system. The parent virus passes on its code to its offspring by giving it copies of its DNA. Once the new virus possesses the code, a bit of nutrient is all that is required to make a whole new virus copy. In other words, once the DNA template (like a plaster mold) is in place, the reproductive process can carry on.

The four nucleosides are each converted to *nucleotides* (discussed later) before they are used to make up the DNA code. Depending on the sequence of nucleotides, the DNA code determines the size of your nose (if it is in your DNA) or the size of your skin sore (if it is in the DNA of your herpes virus). DNA looks much like a helical ladder as it grows (see plate 16, page 102). One side of the ladder is used as the template and is made up of a certain sequence of nucleotides coded according to the first letter of their chemical names: A (adenosine), T (thymidine), G (guanosine), and C (cytosine).

According to the rules of DNA growth and reproduction, there is an exact system, which cannot be altered, for connecting nucleotides (see figure 14 below). The first rule of the system is that A's always get linked side by side to T's; G's always get linked to C's. Thus, in the growth of the DNA ladder depicted in the figure, the first rung on the left pairs G to C, then T to A, then C to G, then A to T. Each nucleotide has a unique shape for linking only with its complementary nucleotide. The new strand is built parallel to its complementary mold—the template strand. As a component of each nucleotide, there are chemically reactive points that are identified as either 3' ("three prime") or 5' ("five prime"). These reactive points make up the sides of the growing DNA ladder.

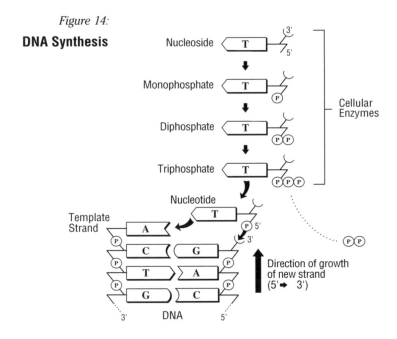

Figure 14:

DNA Synthesis

The second rule of this strict system is that the new strand grows in the 3' direction by tightly interlocking with the last nucleotide in the chain. Chemically, this second rule assures that 5' ends link up to 3' ends so that everything stays oriented with the precision of a military march. The 5' to 3' linkup is orchestrated by *DNA polymerase,* the system's catalyst, which makes sure that the last 3' end finds the next nucleotide in exactly the right orientation, so that it hooks tightly to the 3' end of the next nucleotide, which then exactly complements the opposing nucleotide in the template, and so on.

Acyclovir does not possess a 3' end. In most other ways, however, acyclovir resembles the G (deoxyguanosine) in the linkup system (see plate 16, page 102). In fact, acyclovir was originally called *acycloguanosine,* or *acyclo G.* DNA polymerase picks up the acyclo G thinking it is a real G and successfully links up its 5' end to the 3' end of the growing strand. Following the rules, of course, G is across from C. Continuing in its unyielding and single-minded fashion, DNA polymerase grabs up a new nucleotide to be the next link in the assembly line. In the figure, the new nucleotide is a T brought in to pair up with an A in the template. It takes the 5' end of T and tries to link it up with the 3' end of G. But acyclo G has no 3' end, so no linkup is possible. Acyclo G stops the growth of the DNA chain, as a key broken inside a lock prevents another key from opening the door. This mechanism is called *obligate chain termination.* There are many types of chain termination that may be just as effective although not necessarily obligate. Penciclovir, for example, does possess a 3' end and is therefore not obligate as a chain terminator. However, the shape of the penciclovir molecule does not allow the DNA chain to keep growing once it enters the molecule. This has a very similar effect on the virus but the DNA termination event occurs a few nucleotides further down the chain when the shape of the DNA becomes distorted.

Both acyclovir and penciclovir are able to play a double jeopardy game. Not only do they stop the chain by ruining the new chain while it is being formed, but they also inhibit the enzyme that placed it there—DNA polymerase. DNA polymerase is the chain growth catalyst, the robot that brings the nucleotide pieces together and links them according to the rules. To DNA, then, acyclovir and penciclovir are deadly poisons. Because of their preference for viral DNA, however, they interfere predominantly with viral rather than human DNA growth.

Nucleosides must first be changed into nucleotides before they can be used for making DNA. This is done by special cellular enzymes which attach phosphate molecules to the nucleosides (a process called phosphorylation). Three phosphates (indicated in the figure as PPP) in all must be attached before the nucleotides can be incorporated into DNA. Without three phosphates, the nucleosides just sit there.

Similarly, acyclovir and penciclovir—as nucleoside analogs— just sit there until activated to their triphosphate forms by these enzymes. The first enzyme to get the ball rolling is thymidine kinase or TK. Thymidine kinase obtains the first phosphate for these agents and attaches it, thereby activating the drugs toward their triphosphate forms. Herpes makes a lot of TK. Our own cells don't make much, and what they do make does not readily accomplish this activation step. There is little doubt that the superior ability of herpes TK to activate these agents over human TK is one key reason for their safety and selectivity in killing herpes-infected cells while leaving normal, healthy cells largely unaffected. Activation by herpes TK is depicted in plate 16.

In summary, penciclovir triphosphate and acyclovir triphosphate are the "real" drugs. They are made in high quantity only in cells with herpes infection. Herpes-infected cells are the only ones that are immediately affected by their anti-DNA activity. Acyclovir triphosphate is made mainly and most quickly in virus-infected cells; however, it is not made exclusively in virus-infected cells. Normal human cells do make phosphorylate acyclovir, although only at very, very low levels—almost below our ability to detect the chemical. Penciclovir triphosphate is similarly virus-driven but may also be made without virus in some liver cells. Because the triphosphate form of this drug is very selective as to which DNA it attaches to, no liver harm is done. (In fact, this drug is being used to treat the hepatitis B virus).

There are some differences between penciclovir and acyclovir in their action in the body. As these drugs receive their phosphate groups to become activated, the natural enzyme processes of the body are also degrading them back to their original forms. Acyclovir triphosphate is converted back to acyclovir within an hour or so after treatment, but penciclovir triphosphate persists for up to twenty hours. Herpes TK synthesizes far more penciclovir triphosphate than acyclovir triphosphate. Thus, much more activated penciclovir is made that persists at the DNA site for a much longer time. The flip side, though, is that penciclovir triphosphate is about a hundred times less active than acyclovir triphosphate in inhibiting viral DNA polymerase. The end result of activity against the virus is about the same.

Someday, the subtle biochemical differences between these two agents may be more clearly identified. For now, they are interesting but have no clear clinical significance.

Positive effects of the antiviral medications

First episodes

First episodes of genital herpes have been effectively treated with oral acyclovir. Dr. Yvonne Bryson at UCLA found first episodes to be shortened by 3.0 days in men and 4.2 days in women. More severe (primary) episodes were shortened by 9.0 days in men and 6.2 days in women. The duration of virus shedding (positive cultures) was also reduced. When more severe symptoms were present, acyclovir also reduced pain, lymph node discomfort, urinary discomfort, and general body aches; these symptoms started to improve by day three or four in most people taking acyclovir.

Dr. G. Mertz and coworkers from many centers across the United States and Canada reported a reduction of five days in men and two days in women with full-blown primary infections; this reduction was, statistically speaking, of borderline significance for women. Among patients with nonprimary first episodes of genital herpes, acyclovir reduced the median time to healing by four days, but this reduction also was not statistically significant. Nevertheless, a dramatic reduction in formation of new lesions was highly significant (18 percent compared to 62 percent). Like Dr. Bryson's study, Dr. Mertz showed that virus shedding was shortened in patients receiving oral acyclovir when compared to those receiving placebo (look-alike pills).

Dr. Bryson has followed the patients from this original study for several years. The true primary patients (see chapter 3) who received acyclovir during this study have had significantly fewer episodes of recurrences after the first year of infection. Other investigators have not found this, but they have not looked beyond the first year. Unfortunately, large-scale definitive studies of this possible benefit were never carried out.

The new oral prodrug formulations, valacyclovir and famciclovir, have both been tested in first episodes also. Because of the benefits of acyclovir shown in the early 1980s, it is no longer considered ethical to compare these drugs to placebo for treating first episodes, which may be prolonged and painful in some people. Therefore, both new drugs were compared with oral acyclovir. Both were shown to be essentially identical to acyclovir in achieving more rapid healing and loss of symptoms. So far, the benefit of the new drugs over oral acyclovir for treating first episodes is limited to easier dosing. Acyclovir is given at a dosage of 200-mg tablets five times daily. Valacyclovir was studied at a dosage of 1,000- mg tablets twice daily for first episodes. Although not studied, a dose of 500 mg twice daily is probably effective also. (This dose has been approved by the Australian regulatory authorities). Famciclovir is given at a dosage of 250-mg tablets three times daily. Duration of treatment should probably be seven to ten days for first episodes, although five days may be sufficient. Regardless of which treatment is prescribed, all first episodes should be treated with acyclovir or one of the new oral agents, valacyclovir (Valtrex) or famciclovir (Famvir).

Recent studies in mice have been conducted by Dr. Hugh Field in the United Kingdom. In these trials, animals were infected with herpes and then treated with antiviral medications. All of the current treatments were able to prevent most of the illness in the mice. In these studies, famciclovir treatments went further and prevented latent herpes virus from being established in the ganglia. The mice treated with famciclovir had acquired herpes that, under the conditions of the experiment, could not reactivate to cause subsequent recurrences. It is premature to assume that these experiments mean anything of importance in human beings. The problem with any animal experiment is, of course, that animals react very differently from humans in response to herpes infections and do not absorb or metabolize drugs in exactly the same way. The herpes strains used for infection are also not random clinical samples but rather specific characterized laboratory strains established for this purpose. Further work is needed to figure out whether the findings bear any clinical relevance. All of the drugs need to be tested in this type of model under different types of laboratory conditions. For now, though, it is clear that in some animals, early treatment of herpes makes a long-term difference.

In summary, the oral antivirals work minor wonders in severe first episodes of herpes. They make people feel better faster, although several days are still required for healing, especially during severe primary episodes. Because of the positive effect on urine problems seen with treatment, which occur commonly in first episodes, it is especially worthy of consideration by people with urinary complaints or those having marked discomfort. Because of the reduction in new lesion formation, which might not be apparent right at the beginning of an episode, oral medication should be used in all first episodes of genital herpes as soon as the diagnosis is suspected, unless the episode is very mild and nearly healed when first seen.

Recurrences

Dr. Richard Reichman from the University of Vermont, along with investigators from San Diego, Seattle, Edmonton, and Montreal, reported findings on 250 patients with recurrent genital herpes. Acyclovir was orally administered at a dosage of 200 mg five times per day for five days. Acyclovir-treated recurrences were shorter than placebo-treated recurrences by 0.7 days on average. When patients treated themselves earlier during their warning signs (such as skin tingling or itching), healing times on acyclovir were shorter by 1.0 day on average. Differences were noted between drug and placebo with regard to itching, pain, and other symptoms. This study was confirmed by a similar trial in Europe. The study generally reflects what we see when people use acyclovir in this way. Oral acyclovir, taken as early as possible in a recurrent episode, preferably during the prodrome or warning period, at a dosage of five 200-mg tablets or capsules per day, will shorten the duration of the episode slightly. Many dosage formats that are more convenient are now commonly used—400 mg three times daily, 200 mg four times daily, and so on. Only the 200 mg five times daily dosage was actually studied. In this study, its benefits were statistically significant. However, this method of treatment did not cause lesions to abort, and it did not significantly reduce symptoms. However, a much larger subsequent study did suggest that acyclovir reduces the duration of lesion pain.

Is the cost of oral antivirals worth the benefits received? Clearly, if recurrences are at all frequent, intermittent use of oral antivirals is not the way to go. Chronic daily suppression with these drugs is preferred by people with frequent episodes. In fact, "preferred" is an understatement. Despite this fact, physicians prescribe antiviral medications for intermittent use ten times as often as for prophylaxis. People with frequent recurrences (more than eight or so lesion episodes per year) often become frustrated and give up treatment with this drug if they are treated intermittently based on their symptoms. This is a shame, because these people would find a very high degree of benefit from prophylactic use of one of these drugs which can completely block most recurrences.

If recurrences are infrequent, however, and an intermittent, occasional method of treatment is preferred, several therapeutic options are now available. The new prodrug oral formulations provide extra options.

Valacyclovir (Valtrex) has been extensively studied for treatment of acute recurrent episodes. In a study comparing valacyclovir to acyclovir and placebo, this agent was shown to decrease the duration of sores, the duration of virus shedding from sores, and lesion pain compared with placebo treatment. In a separate study published in the *Archives of Internal Medicine*, Dr. S. L. Spruance and his colleagues confirmed the benefits of valacyclovir against lesion pain and duration and discomfort. In addition, they found a reduction in the proportion of people who used treatment early in the episode who went on to develop vesicles or ulcers of the skin. About 31 percent of people who took the drug did not develop these phases compared with 21 percent of people who took the placebo. This abortive effect has not been seen in every study of valacyclovir, nor does it happen for every person who tries it, but the effect is definitely encouraging. The proper dose of this medicine for recurrent herpes is 500-mg tablets twice daily.

Another new treatment for recurrent genital herpes is famciclovir (Famvir). Studies on famciclovir as treatment for individual recurrent genital herpes episodes from our center and several other Canadian centers, published in the *Journal of American Medical Association*, showed that oral famciclovir, taken at the onset of a prodrome or lesion, significantly lessened the time virus was on the skin and also speeded healing. Famciclovir, when taken early, reduced the number of culture-positive episodes and when taken a bit later reduced the number of culture-positive new lesions. Treatment shortened the vesicle, ulcer, and crust stages and reduced the time required for lesion swelling to go down. Famciclovir also lessened the duration of each of the common uncomfortable symptoms of recurrent genital herpes infections (pain, itch, tenderness) and relieved all symptoms significantly more quickly than placebo. The proper dose of famciclovir for recurrent herpes is 125-mg tablets twice daily. For people who do not require continuous antiviral suppression for frequent recurrences, episodic use of valacyclovir or famciclovir may be worth a try. So far, no studies have directly compared the new treatments with each other. As study designs were different, we can only say, at this point, that each drug was shown to be effective when studied individually. If episodic treatment makes sense to you, the new treatments provide very convenient dosing and good effects on reducing discomfort. They are very nice to have available. You be the judge.

Prophylaxis

Many investigative groups have analyzed the effects of these antiviral agents in preventing recurrent herpes. Although each study has a slightly different design, all have found essentially the same positive results. Dr. Steve Straus at the National Institutes of Health, along with coworkers, studied thirty-five healthy adults with genital herpes. Each participant had a recurrence frequency of more than one episode per month. On average, people receiving acyclovir took 137.7 days to have a recurrence after starting treatment, whereas placebo recipients required an average of about 45 days. After the treatment was stopped, people from both groups got recurrences within a month on average.

The Seattle study reported by Dr. John Douglas and coworkers showed equally impressive results. Participants, all of whom had six recurrences or more in the year before the study, were divided into low-dose (two 200-mg capsules per day) and high-dose (five 200-mg capsules per day) groups. Of 47 placebo recipients, 44 (94 percent) had recurrences during four months of therapy. Of 45 low-dose recipients, 13 (29 percent) had recurrences. Of 51 high-dose recipients, 18 (35 percent) had recurrences. The acyclovir recipients' recurrences were shorter. After the drug was withdrawn, both groups developed recurrences again.

From London, Dr. A. Mindel and associates reported similar findings. Fifty-six patients with at least four episodes per year were given 200 mg or placebo four times per day. The recurrence rate was 1.4 per month in placebo recipients and 0.05 per month in acyclovir recipients. Again, no differences were seen after the drug was withdrawn.

Several other studies have added to acyclovir's impressive record. In an oral acyclovir prophylaxis trial performed simultaneously at my clinic in Vancouver and by Dr. Joe Portnoy in Montreal, volunteers who had at least one episode per month for one year or more each received three capsules of acyclovir 200 mg or placebo every day for six months. If a visible lesion developed during the study, the episode was treated for five days with five capsules per day. During the treatment period, approximately one-third of volunteers receiving acyclovir had no episodes and another one-third had only one episode of visible lesions. The people receiving placebo continued to have their usual (more than one) number of episodes per month. During this study, however, episodes of nonlesional prodromes only (tingling or itching but no visible sore) were more common in the group of acyclovir recipients. Dr. Straus reported similar findings in his study. It is likely that recurrences recycled and began in our study, despite acyclovir prophylaxis. They did so at just about the same rate as without treatement, but in most cases they did not develop into visible sores. Nobody knows if these warnings are associated with shedding of virus from skin. After several months of acyclovir suppression, most nonlesional episodes usually decrease, as if the body finally realizes that it is not getting most of its recurrences. Nevertheless, it would be wise to refrain from genital contact during these "beginnings."

In another study, from the United States, a large number of patients have been followed during chronic treatment for several years to determine acyclovir's continued safety and efficacy. Dr. Greg Mertz reported results from several hundred patients who took acyclovir for one or two years at a dose of 400 mg twice daily. Acyclovir maintained its suppressive effect over this time. Generally, about 25 percent of patients experience a breakthrough recurrence every three to four months. Follow-up studies on this dosage for up to seven years of continuous treatment have now been reported: the safety record over this period remains excellent. The benefits do not really change, either. Once every eight months, on average, there is a mild breakthrough recurrence.

Dr. Anna Wald and her colleagues in Seattle recently examined the effects of oral acyclovir suppression on asymptomatic shedding of virus from the genital tract of women who had recently experienced their first episode of herpes. Previous studies with oral acyclovir for asymptomatic shedding focused on a different group and yielded disappointing results. Dr. Wald's study showed a very clear reduction (but not elimination) of asymptomatic viral shedding because of suppressive treatment in women during the first two years after primary infection. Studies with the other oral antiviral agents are now under way to determine if the effects can be improved even further. Each of the new drugs is likely to have a similar effect, but study results are pending.

Some people try to reduce the dosing of acyclovir to once daily. This is not recommended. I prefer to recommend smaller doses more frequently, because the body absorbs only a small amount of oral acyclovir and clears it from the system very quickly: no matter how high the dose, once daily dosing results in long periods with very little acyclovir circulating in the bloodstream. If you can take pills more frequently, three or four 200-mg tablets spaced out over the day cost the same and give good results. Another convenient dosing format is 400 mg twice daily. This is the usual suppressive dose. Taking 400 mg twice daily costs about the same as taking one 800-mg tablet and is a bit more expensive than taking 200 mg three times daily. Many of my patients use one 200-mg tablet twice daily—a proven and effective dosing regimen that reduces the cost. It would be very interesting to know if the different doses affect the number of breakthroughs or the number of days with asymptomatic shedding, about which little is known.

Studies with famciclovir have also shown a reduction of symptomatic recurrences during suppressive therapy. Dr. G. Mertz and colleagues compared various doses of famciclovir for suppression and found that 250 mg twice daily was a very effective regimen. A subsequent trial presented by Dr. F. Diaz-Mitoma and colleagues confirmed the effectiveness and safety of this dose in people with frequent recurrences. Several additional studies are taking place to extend these studies. Dr. L. Corey and colleagues have shown also that chronic famciclovir use reduces asymptomatic viral shedding in people who have both herpes and AIDS. Similar studies have been conducted in people who have normal immune systems, but results have not yet been announced. Acyclovir and famciclovir have not yet been compared for suppressive treatment.

Valacyclovir has also been studied for use in chronic suppressive therapy and is also very effective. Different doses have been studied, including a once-daily treatment with 500 mg. For convenience, this would be very nice. However, studies comparing different doses have not yet been published. Until we have data showing that once daily treatment is equivalent to twice daily, we should probably stick with a twice daily regimen—especially if one of your reasons for taking chronic suppression is for its beneficial effects on asymptomatic shedding. But keep your mind open here while we await the results of trials. Once daily dosing will be very convenient if that turns out to be an equally effective approach.

In summary, all three antiviral medications, valacyclovir, famciclovir, and acyclovir are effective agents for chronic suppressive therapy. Possible additional benefits of the prodrugs—like improved symptom reduction, fewer breakthroughs, better inhibition of asymptomatic shedding—are all still under investigation.

You should discuss the various options with your physician and come up with the best approach for you at the time you need treatment, given your financial situation, your drug insurance, your memory for pill-taking, the latest results of clinical trials and FDA decisions, and your general attitude about these matters.

What are the side effects of these agents?

Acyclovir has proven to be extremely safe. Taking oral acyclovir does not generally cause blood tests to change at all (except in newborns where white blood cell counts may decrease). The drug does not make you sick in any serious way. In fact, most studies have shown no significant side effects compared with placebo, although the occasional person has developed allergy to acyclovir and has had an allergic skin rash, which cleared up after the person stopped using the medication. Some people taking oral acyclovir get headaches and/or muscle aches, although these effects rarely cause people to stop taking it. Oral acyclovir has been prescribed more than 50 million times in the United States. Almost everyone would agree that its safety record has been remarkably clean.

Some people, when given intravenous acyclovir quickly and at very high doses, have developed acute kidney failure. This problem is avoided by taking the drug slowly and has never been seen after oral treatment. Abnormal effects on the brain such as confusion and decreased consciousness have occasionally been seen in very complicated medical cases involving intravenous use. These effects are probably the result of drug excess caused by kidney problems and similar situations. Since kidney failure is very unlikely to occur with the low doses used for genital herpes, a kidney function test is not considered routine for this.

Acyclovir was discovered about fifteen years ago, so long-term effects in humans are not fully known. Moderately long-term clinical studies have extended to more than six years, however. Dr. Kenneth Fife and colleagues have published their findings in the *Journal of Infectious Diseases* on a group of patients who have for several years taken acyclovir for chronic suppression, including more than 200 patients who have taken oral acyclovir without stopping for seven years. In May 1993, Dr. L. Goldberg and his colleagues published their five-year benchmark data from this group in the *Archives of Dermatology*. No significant problems have developed, to date, with long-term oral use. Chronic suppression continues to be just about as effective and as safe in the later years of taking the medication as it does in the first year. In the past few years, the number of patients taking acyclovir daily has moved into the tens of millions. Sales of acyclovir account for hundreds of millions of dollars per year. (Acyclovir becomes generic in the United States in 1997.) To date, there have been no serious toxicities or irreversible side effects. Nor has there been demonstrated any significant loss of effectiveness of long-term therapy in patients whose immunity is not compromised. This means that if acyclovir is some day shown to be toxic, even in the long term, it will be a very subtle type of toxicity that is very difficult to prove, even epidemiologically. It is probably fair to conclude from the wide clinical experience now available that the potential benefits of treatment generally far outweigh any theoretical risk. Acyclovir studies are now very slowly being extended even into pregnancy. Acyclovir could theoretically provide significant benefits in pregnancy. For example, suppression of recurrent herpes at term would be very likely to remove completely the need for cesarean section in women with recurrent herpes. Use of acyclovir for first episode herpes in pregnancy has been used in many cases, especially in the third trimester. During the long-term studies so far available, no significant side effects have been seen except the minor ones noted above. Furthermore, animals observed after taking this drug have done pretty well on acyclovir and have not had much in the way of side effects. One of the animal side effects seen at very high dosage was a detrimental effect on sperm production in dogs. Human studies performed to look for toxicity identified no significant detrimental effects. There are very few new drugs with such a mild side effects profile. Animals who become pregnant on acyclovir have normal offspring. At high doses (beyond those people use), some animals have become very sick and/or suffered hair loss. These effects have not been seen in people taking the recommended doses of acyclovir. Animals do not have any increased rates of cancer or other mutations, although some breaking of chromosomes (the part of the cells containing the DNA) has been noted in animals receiving very high doses.

Because of oral acyclovir's very clean safety record, its manufacturer, Burroughs Wellcome (now Glaxo Wellcome), asked the United States Food and Drug Administration (FDA) for permission to sell capsules over the counter (without prescription). This request was considered carefully in two expert panel meetings. Several arguments were made by sides. The request was turned down by the FDA, although no serious concerns about side effects were ever raised by the panels.

Valacyclovir and famciclovir are fairly new on the scene, so there are no long-term data available in human beings. However, both of the new agents appear to be very safe in the studies so far conducted. Because valacyclovir becomes acyclovir, it is reasonable to assume that it will be identical in safety with acyclovir. However, the body is exposed to far more drug with either of the new pro-drugs because of their improved absorption. For the occasional person, this could make headaches or nausea more of a problem, but, so far, studies have not identified any serious side effects for any of these drugs. Famciclovir has been studied in animals, as well. In one study of rats, more breast tumors appeared in animals treated with very high doses. This was a subtle finding with unknown significance. Furthermore, it is very hard to compare studies like this because of the large differences in oral absorption between famciclovir and the previous drugs. The animals receive far more drug with famciclovir. In another study of rats, famciclovir had a negative effect on sperm production. Human studies in sperm production, however, have not shown any harmful effects of continuous treatment. To date, all of the current treatments appear to be very safe.

Does resistance to drug treatment develop?

Resistance has become increasingly important over the past few years. More and more virus strains have lost their susceptibility to acyclovir. To date, almost all resistant viral strains that show clinical relevance (sores refusing to heal on treatment) have been obtained from patients with severely compromised immunity from, for example, AIDS or leukemia. There is good reason for this. When a normal host develops a recurrence while taking acyclovir, viral strains inside the lesion begin to develop resistance, but the

239

immune system clears the virus anyway. Latent virus inside the ganglion is usually not affected much by treatment and has not therefore developed resistance, so the resistance does not get the chance to create a clinical situation. By contrast, when a person with AIDS who has very compromised immunity (CD4 counts are usually less than 25 at this point, compared with normal counts of 600 to 1,000) develops a recurrence while taking acyclovir, the episode may persist, because the immune cells for fighting off the infection are not available. Resistance is a three-sided affair, requiring, 1) a high number of viral particles, 2) use of the antiviral, and 3) compromised immunity.

We remain watchful concerning drug resistance. Nobody wants to see the benefit of this important treatment diminished in any way. Two recent publications have raised concern about resistance. First, Dr. Rhonda Kost and colleagues described, in the *New England Journal of Medicine,* a patient with normal immunity whose genital herpes infection was acyclovir-resistant. He had apparently caught resistant herpes from a partner who had compromised immunity. Subsequently, Dr. Ann-Christine Nyquist reported in the *Journal of Pediatrics* the case of an infant with neonatal herpes. This baby also had acyclovir-resistant herpes and, except for being an infant, was not immunocompromised. So the question remains: will herpes become more resistant to acyclovir in the future? So far, we have seen only occasional case reports, but we still have to be very careful. For now, the otherwise healthy host usually does not have acyclovir-resistant herpes. If you are experiencing lots of outbreaks while taking acyclovir, there is probably an explanation for it other than resistance.

There are two basic means by which herpes simplex virus can develop resistance to acyclovir. The first involves the enzyme thymidine kinase (TK), discussed above. Since acyclovir is not activated without TK, if the virus loses its TK, it also loses its susceptibility to acyclovir. This type of change develops readily in the laboratory setting and has also been seen to partially develop in some patients during acyclovir oral prophylaxis of genital herpes. Because acyclovir does not really have any effect on latent infection in the ganglion, however, this altered resistance does not seem to be permanent. In other words, resistance may reduce the effectiveness of acyclovir on one recurrence, but so far this has not been a permanent change. Next recurrence, the virus, which starts fresh from the ganglion, is usually susceptible to acyclovir once again. Recent studies have begun to show longer persistence of acyclovir resistant strains in patients who are severely immunocompromised. A recent report from investigators at the National Institutes of Health has also confirmed the fact that resistant virus can be transmitted to another person and can establish a new latent infection in a nonimmunocompromised host. While this event is very rare, the fact that it can occur suggests that we need to keep a strong surveillance on the risks of resistance developing in the future—even in otherwise normal patients with no immunocompromising disease.

The second mechanism of resistance to acyclovir results from changes in the viral DNA polymerase. Clinically, only two instances of resistance from mutations of the viral DNA polymerase have occurred. Both people had severe immune problems. A task force on herpes resistance has now been established through grants from Glaxo Wellcome, Inc. The Centers for Disease Control are also surveying clinics all over the United States to determine how common resistance really is.

What if I have symptoms of herpes while taking medication? Does that mean my herpes has become resistant?

A word of caution. People with herpes who are normal hosts taking any of the oral antiviral agents develop breakthrough episodes of recurrent herpes. True breakthrough recurrences of herpes during suppressive treatment are generally quite mild. They usually consist of small outbreaks that last only a couple of days but shed virus nevertheless. These episodes are just like regular culture-proven untreated herpes, only milder. In some cases, they become frequent. For such people, a significant increase in the dose of acyclovir may be required, or it may be better to switch to one of the prodrugs. As long as these typical episodes heal up quickly, there is no need for alarm. Talk to your physician about changing the medication. This does not mean your immunity is compromised. Even more common is the person, most often (but not exclusively) female, who experiences almost continuous "outbreaks" despite taking one of these medications. This can be extremely frustrating and even frightening for people who expect great relief from treatment, commit themselves to the cost and proper dosing, and find that they are experiencing irritation anyway. The vast majority of these people do not have any immunity problem or resistance to drugs. Most people with herpes who have frequently recurrent or nonhealing skin irritations on the genitals while taking suppressive therapy have something other than herpes. In fact, this method of therapy is so effective that it can almost be considered a small clinical trial to determine whether or not you have more than herpes. Sometimes, whatever else is causing this irritation or skin breakdown is easily diagnosed and treated. For example, vulvar yeast infections, which are often easily treated with antifungal agents, sometimes require chronic intermittent dosing with an antifungal, many of which are now available as topical over-the-counter medications. However, there are many causes of chronic vulvar irritation other than herpes and yeast. You should notify your physician if you are continuing to have genital skin irritation after being treated with suppressive therapy. The cause should be determined, or, at the very least, treatable and/or serious causes should be excluded. If you are having recurrences fairly regularly while taking medication you should go to the physician for confirmation that what you have is truly herpes. Usually, viral culture is the preferred method for determining this.

There are other common reasons for treatment failure. Most physicians prescribe treatments for individual episodes. Some of the recent advances in treatment support this approach, but for people with frequent recurrences of herpes, repeats of the outbreak-treatment cycle can be very frustrating and costly. Most people with frequent herpes will find a far better result from using one of the oral antiviral agents on a suppressive basis. In other words, people in that category should take medication at least twice daily (and evenly-spaced doses), based on the calendar, not on the symptoms. You decide when you would like your herpes to be suppressed or not based on medical, lifestyle, and personal decisions.

Are there any other problems with taking medication?

A quick word about antibodies. Antibodies help to heal active herpes sores and may help to prevent some people from getting sores in the first place. The body triggers itself to make antibodies in its own defense, so any drug that minimizes the amount of virus on the attack will cause a decreased counterresponse. Thus, Drs. Ashley and Corey found that only 30 percent of people receiving intravenous acyclovir made one specific virus antibody, vp66, while all people receiving placebo made this antibody within the first thirty days of their primary. If people did not make it on the first go-round, they made vp66 and the other antibodies on their first recurrence. Drs. D. Bernstein, M. Lovett, and Y. Bryson from UCLA have published similar findings in a study of oral acyclovir, in which the quantity of neutralizing antiherpes antibody was reduced by treatment.

Since reduction of immunity is probably the result of decreasing the virus load on the immune system, these observations almost certainly do not indicate any problem. Perhaps future therapy will include both vaccines and treatments. So far, antibody reduction in itself is probably not a reason to avoid suppressive therapy.

Should I or shouldn't I?

It goes without saying that you are the only person who can make up your mind. Although ultimately it is a personal choice, you should decide in conjunction with your physician. In preparation for discussions with him or her, it is useful to weigh the benefits and risks in order to help you decide if taking oral antiviral treatment is worth it for you.

On the positive side, oral antiviral agents taken prophylactically do markedly and predictably reduce episode frequency. Data also show that they reduce the rates of asymptomatic shedding dramatically. These drugs have few, if any, significant short-term side effects. At prescribed doses for up to seven years (the period studied so far) long-term safety with acyclovir has been demonstrated.

On the negative side, these medications work by inhibiting DNA. The inhibition of DNA occurs almost exclusively, but not totally exclusively, in virus-infected cells. Because they are effective only when taken internally, it is not possible to deliver drugs only to the areas that need it on the skin. Because of their virus-dependent mechanism of action, these oral antiviral medications are chemically directed to the affected areas, in part because the active DNA inhibitor is synthesized preferentially inside cells that are infected with herpes. So far, animal tests, human clinical trials, and widespread clinical use over acyclovir's first several years have shown an excellent record of safety in adults. Use in children also appears to be safe (see pages 152–155) but treatment in any setting—especially in infants or children—requires that a physician weigh with the parents the possible benefits and risks. Treatment with any prescription medication should never be undertaken without the specific prescription of a professional. Oral acyclovir is currently used by hundreds of thousands of people every day. With a few exceptions at very high doses in animals, the predictive factors for all of these drugs are good ones. Long-term safety has been very well established for acyclovir after five to seven years of consistently good reports in adults with genital herpes. In earlier editions of this book, I used strong caution in advising people to consider using treatment only in the most necessary cases. After seeing a pristine record in patients, however, I now feel acyclovir's good safety record justifies its use in many more situations. So far, the newer prodrugs also look very clean, but clinical experience is not as extensive simply because they are new. In many situations, however, they may offer advantages that you want to consider. People should not use this drug if they do not need it or would not benefit from it. However, if you want to decrease lesion frequency and can afford this drug, you should be aware that its safety track record, to date, is excellent.

What are the theoretical concerns about these drugs? There are three major areas of concern about changes in DNA: teratogenesis (birth defects), oncogenesis (cancer), and mutagenesis (mutations). All three have been and continue to be carefully studied. So far, tests continue to suggest that all these agents are safe. In humans, none of these agents have been adequately tested in the setting of pregnancy. The manufacturers recommend that they should not be taken during pregnancy, especially early pregnancy. You should avoid becoming pregnant until several weeks after stopping any of these drugs, unless you and your physician have decided to use treatment in pregnancy for some specific benefit. These agents are pretty much cleared from the system within a day of stopping treatment, but if minute quantities were sticking around in cells, they would not be detected by the tests presently available. There is no evidence, to date, of any increase in birth defects or other problems in women who have taken acyclovir in pregnancy. This is quite different, however, from saying that acyclovir is *safe* in pregnancy, since that has not yet been *proven*. You may wish to refer further to page 152. These are decisions that can only be made between a pregnant woman and her doctor, since special situations may apply. In fact, acyclovir's safety is considered high enough that some studies are now being conducted in which this drug is being tried as a herpes suppressant during late pregnancy (see chapter 6). In certain situations, such as true primary genital herpes in late pregnancy or chickenpox pneumonia in pregnancy, many physicians may choose to use acyclovir during pregnancy. But there are still very few pregnancy "experiences" on the prodrugs on which to base an intelligent clinical decision.

Before you decide whether you should take any of these medicines, it is important to decide if they might benefit you. If you are having a painful primary episode with swollen glands, difficulty with urination, headache, etc., a seven to ten-day (or even five-day) course of oral acyclovir or famciclovir or valacyclovir will definitely make you feel better up to one week earlier! Because of this, using oral treatment during a first episode, as early as possible, is definitely a good idea. By contrast, if you have one mild recurrence of genital herpes per year, continuous treatment would be of minimal use to you. You will greatly benefit from taking one of the antiviral medicines if one of the following descriptions applies to you:

1. You are having a first episode, especially with lesion pain or lymph node pain requiring pain relief or with problems urinating or headache. You would use 200 mg of acyclovir five times per day, valacyclovir 500 to 1,000 mg twice per day (although untested, 500 mg is probably an effective dose and is approved in Australia), or famciclovir 250 mg three times per day for seven to ten days.

2. You are having frequent recurrent herpes episodes that you are sure are herpes each time (not chronic yeast infections, for example), and this frequency rate has been sustained for quite

a while (say, six months to a year or more). The episodes are bothersome.

Under these circumstances, you could try one 200-mg capsule or tablet of acyclovir two or three times a day up to two 200-mg capsules or tablets (or one 400-mg capsule or tablet) twice per day. That dose—400 mg twice daily—is the one used in the longest term U.S. studies on continuing safety. The suppressive dose of famciclovir is 250 mg twice daily. A study recently reported from the United Kingdom supports the use of valacyclovir 500 mg once daily as an effective suppressive dose in reducing recurrences. More studies need to be done, however, to prove that a single daily dose can be as effective as twice daily doses against both symptomatic recurrences, as well as asymptomatic shedding. Nevertheless, if a single daily suppressive treatment turns out to be just as effective as twice daily, this will make continuous suppressive therapy more convenient. In general, it is wise to space your doses evenly, so that a twice-daily dose is taken every twelve hours, a three-times-a-day dose every eight hours, and so on. You can expect that the vast majority of your lesional recurrences should be thwarted by suppressive treatment at any of the doses described, although you may still get tingles or other warnings, which you should, for now, consider to be short recurrences. They will probably disappear, for the most part, after six months or so of continuous suppressive treatment. Suppression is effective in preventing both type 1 and type 2 herpes infections on all skin areas.

Once you stop these drugs, you should expect to get sores at about the same frequency as before. Some people find that the sores come more often or feel slightly different in the period right after they stop treatment, but most people find that the sores are just the same as before. If convenient, you may wish to limit your periods of prophylaxis to those where you need to be free of lesions. These are physical, emotional, and lifestyle decisions which you can make with the advice of your doctor.

3. You have recurrent genital herpes that is not frequent enough for you to wish to take continuous treatment. You have considered continuous treatment's potential benefit of reduced asymptomatic shedding. You wish to now treat individual episodes to get symptomatic and lesion relief more quickly than nature provides on its own. Famciclovir studies have shown that treatment early in the episode reduces the times to healing and crusting as well as the duration of all of the active phases of infection and all of the uncomfortable symptoms. In some people, famciclovir also reduces the formation of new culture-positive episodes and lesions depending on how early in the episode it is taken. Valacyclovir studies have also shown a reduction in the time required for lesions of herpes to heal as well as the time required for pain and discomfort to disappear. In one study, valacyclovir reduced the proportion of patients who went on to develop blisters or ulcers.

You may wish to try either or both of these treatments (not at the same time). Both agents offer a new, more convenient approach to the episodic treatment of individual recurrences. Both are safe and effective at reducing the durations of lesions, virus, and discomfort. Because they have never been compared directly, it is not possible to recommend one over the other. Discuss the issues with your doctor and look at what each has shown in studies and what you wish to accomplish through treatment.

4. You have recurrent herpes as well as moderate to severe eczema. I would advise chronic suppressive treatment here because of the risk of autoinoculation of herpes to areas of involved skin. If outbreaks of herpes are infrequent, you may wish to use either valacyclovir or famciclovir as soon as you have a warning of an outbreak. Oral acyclovir at a dose of 200 mg five times daily has also shown some benefits for the treatment of individual episodes.

5. Erythema multiforme, which is sometimes caused by herpes, should (when it is thought to be triggered by herpes) be treated with antiviral medication either chronically or intermittently, depending on the frequency rate. If treatment does not fully

prevent the skin rash, your doctor may want you to take other medication as well.

6. If you have AIDS and herpes, you should probably be taking oral antiviral medications as a suppressive regimen to avoid serious complications. The same is true for other types of immunocompromise, such as leukemia and transplantation. Your doctor can guide you about when you should take treatment.

What if your recurrent herpes is neither frequent nor severe? Then your choice about whether to use oral treatment falls into a gray zone, and you will have to reach your own decision after considering the facts:

1. Treating mild first episodes of herpes. The less severe the problem, the less the gain from treatment. However, early in a first clinical episode, neither the physician nor the patient can accurately determine whether or not an episode is a true primary. A single mild sore could develop into a serious primary after a few days. Thus, unless the physician can instantly perform the antibody test required to differentiate primary from nonprimary initial episodes, treatment with an oral antiviral should probably be begun as soon as possible.

2. Preventing less frequent herpes recurrences by daily prophylaxis. What is the cutoff? Obviously, daily systemic treatment to prevent one episode a year is not worth it. Usually, preventing three episodes per month is worth it. A generally held cutoff is one recurrence every four to six weeks. In some cases, as few as four to six episodes per year will be a reasonable cutoff. Eight to twelve recurrences per year definitely warrants consideration for chronic suppression. If you gain five days of being lesion-free for every fifty, this represents only 10 percent of the time. Five days for every hundred days is a gain of 5 percent, and so on. It's tempting to take a pill and feel one is regaining control of one's condition, but consider what your control will gain for you. Even taking antivirals every day does not usually prevent all outbreaks or totally eliminate the possibility of shedding of virus and has not yet been studied to

see if it may alter the possibility of transmitting the virus to a sexual partner. However, beneficial and dramatic effects in reducing asymptomatic shedding are clear.

3. Preventing outbreaks during special events. Oral antiviral suppression offers control over herpes when you need it. Let's say you only get one outbreak every couple of months, but you are just beginning a new relationship, or experiencing an unusual amount of stress at work, or due for your first vacation in two years, or whatever scenario fits. If you use antivirals for special events, take it as for suppression—i.e., before an outbreak has begun, for a predetermined length of time. When the event is over, you can stop using whatever agent you have chosen.

4. You may consider treatment if your occupation requires it. For example, if you get fairly frequent whitlows (finger infections) and you are a bartender, a dentist, a grocery clerk, a brain surgeon, or an aid in a newborn nursery, antiviral suppression may keep you employed.

5. Preventing herpes in someone who has never had it is not discussed in the drug monograph since this use has not been tested. Yet it will be tempting. Should you allow yourself to be tempted? Antivirals may, in some people, prevent herpes infections after transmission has occurred and before latent infection has been established. It has done so in some animals tested. Treatment has definitely failed to do so in some clinical cases, and (see treatment of first episodes earlier in this chapter) has probably succeeded in some. If you realize after you have had sexual contact that you have a wet lesion in an active phase, you could discuss with your partner the possibility that he or she might use antiviral medication for five or ten days in the hope of preventing infection. If your partner has never had herpes and exposure was fairly certain, he or she may wish to try it. Taking antivirals after transmission has occurred but before symptoms have developed is untested and unproven. While I cannot recommend this approach on the basis of scientific evidence, the risk-to-benefit ratio may be very much in favor of treatment, depending on the situation. Talk to your physician.

What about my unaffected partner taking a treatment all the time?

This is *not* recommended, although one can imagine that it will be tried. Treatment may not even work for this purpose, and chronic exposure to any drug without any evidence of infection is unwise. In this situation, the risk-to-benefit ratio would probably not be in your favor.

Personal conclusions about oral antiviral treatments

It is a great relief to have in one's medicine cabinet a selection of medicines to manage a nagging, persisting, uncomfortable problem. There is no cure available, but the ability to treat first episodes successfully and to treat and prevent herpes recurrences is exciting news. Nevertheless, before taking treatment every day for the next ten years, determine for certain that you are likely to benefit from treatment. If you have carefully reviewed treatment options by reading about them and discussing them with your health care provider, if you feel your problem will likely benefit from treatment, and if you can afford the financial cost, then it is reasonable to proceed with a trial of treatment.

What does the future hold?

The field of drug therapy against herpes has progressed rapidly over the past few years. In 1982, the first proven effective therapy for primary genital herpes—topical acyclovir—gained government approval and appeared in drugstores. By 1985, oral acyclovir was available by prescription. The number of herpes researchers around the world has increased dramatically, possibly more rapidly than the incidence of the infection itself. Pharmaceutical firms have joined in the herpes battle, each one hoping for a chance to have the best therapy for herpes.

Many methods—drugs, chemicals, natural substances, food additives, solvents, biofeedback, hypnosis, acupuncture, and so forth—have been purported to work against herpes. Of the drugs tested in carefully designed double-blind, placebo-controlled, randomized clinical trials, only a handful show any positive effects. (These drugs and some others will be discussed further.)

Any infection results from an imbalance between the number of infecting particles (the invasion size) and the immune defense network. Drugs for herpes are being developed to affect both sides of the balance: drugs can boost the body's natural defenses, so that the body can prevent itself from becoming infected by killing the virus faster or keeping it latent more effectively, or they can actively kill the virus, as penicillin kills gonorrhea.

In the late 1990s, we will see further major advances in the prevention and treatment of genital herpes. Drugs of significantly increasing potency will seek to reduce further asymptomatic viral shedding and asymptomatic disease transmission. Vaccines that boost immunity to specific viral proteins are now under development. Eventually vaccines may be combined with treatments for prevention and recurrence reduction.

Other drugs to kill the virus (antiviral agents)

Phosphonoformic acid (foscarnet, Foscavir)

Foscarnet is a small chemical that works by very different mechanisms from those of the nucleoside analogs. It does not depend on TK at all. Rather, it gets into all kinds of cells, infected or not. Foscarnet is also an enzyme inhibitor. The enzyme it interrupts is DNA polymerase, which tells the four nucleosides to start building the DNA chain. Herpes has its own DNA polymerase, and cells have their own. Foscarnet is a much more potent inhibitor of viral DNA polymerase than of cellular DNA polymerase. This drug was tested in Sweden, where it was shown to decrease the time that lesions were not healed in recurrent herpes from five days to four days. This effect was seen more in men than in women. In this study, women also healed faster, but the differences were not statistically significant. Side effects were observed in men at a cream concentration of one percent. These adverse effects included irritation and occasional ulceration at the site of drug application.

Adverse effects have been avoided by reducing the drug's concentration in the cream. A Canadian study in seven centers showed a good antiviral effect in men. Symptoms were slightly reduced after the first day of treatment. However, the times to healing and the duration of symptoms, overall, were not improved. This outcome demonstrates the need for large, well defined studies before conclusions are drawn about any new agent.

Despite its ineffectiveness as a topical agent, however, intravenous foscarnet is very potent against herpes simplex virus. In most cases, people with herpes do not need an intravenous drug, but in the case of resistant herpes, where a patient with compromised immunity (for example, in AIDS) develops severe and progressive infection despite acyclovir, foscarnet's unique mechanism of action provides a major advantage. Since thymidine kinase is not needed to activate foscarnet, and since most herpes simplex virus becomes resistant by losing thymidine kinase activity and thus the ability to activate the drug, foscarnet provides an alternative. Studies have shown this drug to be a very effective alternative for treating resistant herpes simplex infection. In cases of compromised hosts with resistant infection, foscarnet can literally be life saving. The dose is managed by the physician, since this drug is given in the hospital, and there are significant side effects. However, where herpes is clearly resistant and immunity is compromised, the benefits outweigh the side effects. Side effects are generally avoidable and are manageable if they do occur.

Recent studies have shown that some herpes simplex viral strains that affect people with severely compromised immunity are resistant to both acyclovir and foscarnet. Resistance is possible when the body's immune defenses are unable to help the drug eliminate the virus.

Nucleotide (nucleoside phosphonate) compounds

A chemist from Czechoslovakia, Antonin Holy, and a biologist from Belgium, Erik De Clercq, have teamed up to test an interesting new series of antiviral agents that essentially combine the structures of the acyclovir type and the foscarnet type into one molecule. One of the combinations they have studied, known as cidofovir (Vistide) (a nucleotide analog of the nucleoside, cytosine), was recently approved as a treatment for cytomegalovirus, which is one of the nastiest complications of AIDS. Cidofovir is also very potent against herpes simplex virus. Like penciclovir's, cidofovir's fully phosphorylated form has a long persistence in infected cells.

Cidofovir's persistence seems to be very, very long—possibly as long as several days. Both studies from Europe and the United States show sores caused by herpes simplex virus that is fully resistant to acyclovir can be effectively treated with cidofovir applied as a topical gel (Forvade). Cidofovir is very potent against genital herpes in animals. These nucleotide analogs are not cures. Many new antiviral treatments which can be classified as nucleotide drugs are under development against a wide variety of diseases including herpes. One percent cidofovir gel for now should probably be used only in cases where resistance to acyclovir, valacyclovir, or famciclovir is thought to be truly present and where the person requiring treatment has compromised immunity. This agent is very strong and should not be used as a topical replacement for people with uncomplicated herpes infections until further work has been done. We will be seeing a lot more of antiviral nucleotides in the future.

n-Docosanol

(Lidakol, behenyl alcohol) is a 22-carbon straight chain fatty alcohol. A 10 percent topical antiviral cream formulation has been studied in oral herpes simplex virus infections (cold sores). This agent is a chemical relative of a number of products commonly found in cosmetics. *n*-Docosanol exerts antiviral activity against many enveloped viruses. It has a completely different mechanism of action than other current antiviral agents. It seems to enter the cell membrane and alter it, thus blocking the ability of viruses to enter the cell. Early studies in people showed that the cream was very well tolerated and further suggested a possible clinical benefit. Large, placebo-controlled trials however, failed to demonstrate a reduction in the signs or symptoms of recurrences.

Immunity boosters

Interferon

You may have heard of interferon when it was thought to be a miracle cure for cancer. Interferon originally got its name, in 1957, because it "interfered" with viruses. It has become reasonably inexpensive to make using recombinant DNA tricks.

Results of clinical trials using systemic interferon for genital herpes have shown conflicting results. In general, the side effects are too severe to warrant its general use. Use of interferon in a gel preparation, however, is not associated with significant side effects. In a multicenter study reported in 1987, topical high-dose recombinant interferon had a good antiviral effect and some clinical benefit in the treatment of recurrent herpes. Studies of topically applied interferon combined in a cream with the spermicidal agent nonoxynol-9 also showed some promise. In a study from Vancouver published in the *Journal of Infectious Diseases* in 1990, high-dose topical interferon applied three times daily was found to be effective at reducing the duration of viral shedding from sores by about one and one-half days. The antiviral effects were more prominent in men than in women. People treated with high-dose interferon were found to have a reduction in the duration of symptoms by about one day, and while the effects on healing were not found to reach statistical significance, there was a benefit that approached statistical significance of about 0.7 day. Like edoxudine, this topical antiviral has a demonstrable though small benefit. Approval for this indication is doubtful by government agencies.

Inosiplex

Inosiplex (Isoprinosine) has a direct antiherpes effect in the test tube. It has also been shown to increase lymphocyte transformation against herpes simplex virus. In other words, lymphocytes (see chapter 2) in people receiving this drug get more excited and more active around herpes than they do in people not receiving inosiplex.

In 1972 Drs. Steinberg and Ruiz reported the results of a double-blind, controlled study that showed that herpes sores of people receiving inosiplex healed in 5.2 days as opposed to 9.0 days for placebo recipients' sores. Both oral and genital herpes were studied, but not separately. Primary and recurrent herpes were not kept separate in their analysis. Furthermore, virus cultures were not routinely performed to document herpes infection.

The next year, a report by Drs. Chang, Fuimara, and Weinstein suggested that inosiplex could be useful in primary herpes. Their double-blind, placebo-controlled trial did not suggest any effect on recurrent herpes or on the rate of recurrences. In 1975, Drs. Wickett and Bradshaw concluded, from a double-blind, placebo-controlled study of fifty-three patients, that this drug shortens the course of a herpes outbreak. The most critical design error possible was present in this study: people with primary and recurrent herpes were analyzed together. Of course, primary herpes may last for up to three weeks as compared to five or six days for recurrent herpes. Twice as many primary patients were included in the placebo group. In other words, the people expected to have longer outbreaks had their outbreaks averaged in with the placebo results.

Another study, from Paris, suggested that inosiplex may be effective in recurrent herpes. Lesions dried up by day three in over 50 percent of the drug recipients and only 25 percent of placebo recipients. In a letter to the editor of *The Lancet,* Dr. M. Galli reported the results of giving inosiplex to thirty-one people with genital herpes for one week on four separate occasions. Herpes recurrences declined from the year before treatment, but this effect could not be attributed to the influence of the drug.

Subsequent studies by A. Mindel and others by G. Kinghorn compared acyclovir to isoprinosine. In these controlled trial conditions, acyclovir was effective and inosine was not.

This agent has so far been associated with one side effect: the elevation of uric acid levels in the blood. Uric acid is a metabolite of the drug (a breakdown product) and this elevation is not surprising nor especially worrisome.

Some trials have left more questions than answers. The results of properly controlled trials, however, are not positive. For now, inosiplex should not be used for herpes.

Vaccines

Herpes vaccines have been around for a while. In some European countries, vaccines (for example, Lupidon-G) are available. There has always been some concern about their safety, because herpes in a killed form, such as that present in the vaccine, still has its DNA. There is a theoretical danger that a DNA-containing vaccine might induce cancer, or that a live and attenuated vaccine might revert back to a virulent form and cause infection. Despite these reservations, many people are attracted to whole-virus vaccines because they have a reported capability to induce a 70 to 80 percent improvement rate in frequency and severity of recurrences. These studies were not controlled and are not generally accepted, however. There are no good data on risks with this vaccine. Because there is no proven positive effect and no proven safety record, the vaccine is not approved in the United States or Canada.

Scientists have also discovered ways of deleting specific parts of herpes simplex virus. When certain glycoproteins from the viral envelope are removed, herpes is rendered incapable of reactivating from latency. Such highly engineered viruses cause infection and form latent infection just like the usual clinical strain of herpes, but once infection is complete, there is no potential for recurrences. Such products may become useful as vaccines, since they would induce immunity in the body without causing recurrent infection. Tests in humans have not been conducted, however.

Recently, a great deal of progress has been made toward finding which specific components of the virus are important in stimulating immunity. A successful vaccine must act enough like a real herpes infection that the body responds against it as if it were truly infected. When the body is infected with herpes simplex virus, it responds with a number of different defenses, including cellular defenses and antibody defenses. A potent vaccine might fool the body into making one or all of these defenses. If the defense is strong enough, it might prevent or at least reduce the likelihood of a real infection later. Certain parts of the herpes simplex virus envelope that induce immunity, known as glycoproteins, can be highly purified and given as a vaccine, thereby avoiding injection of viral DNA. Vaccines containing the viral glycoproteins gB and/or gD have been tested in clinical trials. Glycoprotein vaccines have been greatly improved in the past few years by the addition of adjuvants—delivery vehicles that improve the way the viral protein is exposed to the body's immune system. Adjuvants help to stimulate the immune system to react strongly against the glycoprotein. At least two major vaccine companies are investigating glycoprotein vaccine products. One of the major vaccine developers, Chiron-Biocine, has studied the transmission of genital herpes by examining Western blot tests in partners and has announced that their gBgD vaccine product is not effective to prevent genital herpes in partners. Does that mean that vaccines will not be effective for genital herpes? It is far too soon to give up this important search. A specific vaccine product could fail in scientific testing because of the product itself or because the immune-boosters with the product were not strong enough. Vaccine research remains very important and much has been learned from the studies so far that will allow for leads to future candidates. In the meantime, another glycoprotein vaccine containing gD and a strong immune stimulator is still under study both as a potential treatment and as a prevention tool. There are no data available at press time to comment on its effectiveness, but work is continuing on this product worldwide.

Herpes vaccines, if one turns out to be effective, could become very important in the whole field of genital herpes. There are three major areas where the ideal vaccine of the future might become useful:

1. To prevent infection in people at risk of getting genital herpes. If vaccines become successful at prevention, everybody may want to be vaccinated. For now, despite recent setbacks, it is essential that we continue to search for an effective vaccine product that offers protection from infection. People at the greatest risk of getting herpes who might be candidates would include people whose sole sexual partner has genital herpes and who are still susceptible (see chapter 4) and people who are having sexual contact with different partners, especially if sex is unprotected. Herpes vaccines effectively protect animals *before* infection.

2. Pregnant women at risk of acquiring herpes during pregnancy and infants at risk of acquiring herpes during birth. The newborns at greatest risk are born to mothers who have primary genital herpes (see chapter 6). If herpes were to develop in someone who had immunity because of a vaccine, that herpes would probably not act like a primary infection, since the body's immune system would already be prepared.

3. People with recurrent genital herpes who take a vaccine as an immune boost from the extra protein that is specifically targeted at stimulating the immune system. But why should any vaccine be useful to treat recurrent herpes? As far as we can tell, people with herpes have normal amounts of antibody and normal lymphocyte responses to herpes, so what would vaccine-induced increases in immunity accomplish? Would vaccines alter the course of recurrences? Early studies using a gD protein (Chiron-Biocine) suggested that this vaccine was in fact capable of inducing a reduction in recurrence rates without the use of acyclovir suppression. Initial studies published in *The Lancet* by Dr. S. Straus's group at the National Institutes of Health and Dr. L. Corey's group at the University of Washington found that the rate of outbreaks per month was lowered to four per year in people who received the gD vaccine compared with six per year in people who received the placebo. Unfortunately, follow-up studies with a more potent vaccine have not confirmed these early findings.

Vaccines and drug treatments may be used together in the future if studies with more potent vaccines show promise. Patients may be vaccinated to boost their immunity while partners are vaccinated to reduce their risk of infection. Because herpes can develop in some people who already are immune, vaccine will probably not be an absolute preventative, but it may make transmission more difficult. Of course, if all children are vaccinated, they may grow up without a significant genital herpes risk at all. New vaccines under development enhance special components of the immune system. Advances in vaccine engineering are occurring rapidly.

What are the alternative treatments?

Until recently, with the advent of new and effective specific anti-herpes drug therapy, alternatives to drugs were the only forms of treatment available. Now there are several very safe drugs that have been proven effective for the treatment of herpes and, as discussed above, a number of very important advances are likely to come along soon. Alternative treatments are generally not as effective as the proven ones. Thus, you should give the alternative route very careful thought before embarking on it, especially if by choosing it you would be keeping yourself from receiving a treatment known to be effective.

Some of the alternative chemicals listed here are not drugs in the legal sense. A drug has to undergo rigorous testing before it is allowed to be licensed and sold for physicians to prescribe. In order to gain the license, the drug must be shown to be effective in the treatment of the disease for which it is being recommended and safe enough that the benefits of treatment outweigh the risks. Alternative drugs and chemicals do not have to meet these criteria. Some reasons that alternative chemicals may remain available are as follows:

1. The chemical was given drug status before government control came into effect—i.e., the "grandfather clause" applies.

2. The chemical is considered safe without testing because it is a food by-product. An example is L-lysine, in some countries; in others it is not available.

3. The chemical is considered safe because it is an accepted food additive. BHT is an example.

4. The chemical is licensed by a government in another country and is imported for personal use.

The fact that you are able to buy a chemical that someone says you can take as medicine does not necessarily mean that anyone knows it is safe or effective. It is only tested for safety and efficacy if it is called a drug and taken through drug clearance channels. BHT and L-lysine, among others, have never been shown to be safe or effective in humans in the doses recommended by some people for herpes. Nevertheless, just like drugs in the pharmacy, these chemicals go into the body, circulate in the blood, deposit in body tissue, and so on.

The list of potential alternative treatments for herpes is very long. Alternative treatments may involve potential dangers. For example, if ineffective alternatives are sought in lieu of proven treatments for a life-threatening but potentially curable disease, needless deaths may result. Of course, this is not the case with herpes, because herpes is not normally life-threatening. But pursuing ineffective treatments because they may seem more "natural" or less expensive can victimize people and cause significant harm because they can rob people of money, time, and even hope. Standard therapies used incorrectly can do the same, of course. Be selective and careful when choosing alternative or standard therapies. The alternatives arousing the greatest interest are listed below. This is not intended to be a complete list.

Butylated hydroxy toluene (BHT)

BHT is a food additive that is synthesized from two organic compounds called *p-cresol* and *isobutylene.* It cannot be dissolved in water but is easily dissolved in organic solvents such as alcohol and gasoline. BHT is literally everywhere. In 1976, Americans consumed, by mouth, nearly nine million pounds of the stuff. BHT hides in margarine, instant potatoes, and chewing gum, to mention only a few examples. It is fed to chickens and other animals. Americans consume 1 to 2 mg each per day. Each American has on the average 1.3 ± 0.82 parts per million in body fat.

BHT kills herpes simplex virus in the laboratory. When dissolved in mineral oil at a concentration of 5 percent or 15 percent and applied to the skin of hairless mice infected with herpes simplex virus type 1, BHT is better than mineral oil alone at reducing the number of herpes lesions. BHT is probably a virus envelope interrupter: it probably kills viruses that depend on having an envelope by dissolving the envelope. Other mechanisms are also possible. Two important criteria in drug testing have been satisfied in the testing of BHT as an antiherpes treatment:

1. It kills herpes simplex virus in the test tube.

2. It is effective at speeding the healing of sores in mice when applied to the skin in mineral oil, although not all investigators agree.

As a topically applied mixture in mineral oil, BHT therapy also resulted in skin reddening and some skin sloughing. This agent has never been reported to have been given by mouth to animals for treatment of herpes. Despite this, it was extensively advanced by a book that was very popular in the 1980s, at doses ranging from 250 mg to 2,000 mg per day in the treatment of herpes. There are no published data anywhere in the scientific literature on the safety of BHT administered in these doses to humans. Because we take BHT every day as a food additive, it is presumed safe. However, these doses are as much as 1,000 times the usual daily intake. At even higher doses, the following things happen to animals in experiments (not a complete list):

- Mice given an otherwise improper and incomplete synthetic diet lived longer if the diet was supplemented with BHT.
- BHT did not affect the life span of mice who were given proper nutrition, although it did seem to partially reverse the hazardous effects of inadequate nutrition.
- BHT prolonged the life span of mice whose diets began to be supplemented with BHT when they were eleven weeks old. It was of less benefit if started earlier in life.
- At higher doses, it can cause animals to bleed into the brain or even bleed to death.
- It can damage heart cells.
- It can retard weight gain.
- It can decrease the metabolism of the adrenal glands.
- It can cause disorganization and destructive changes of lung cells and can lead to serious lung damage.
- The liver becomes enlarged, a phenomenon that disappears when the agent is stopped. A system of liver enzymes called the P-450 system is induced. If this system stays induced for long periods, it changes the way other drugs and natural products are metabolized. For example, if vitamin D is metabolized more quickly by induced enzymes, over a period of time a vitamin deficiency may develop that can lead to a bone disease called osteomalacia.

Most of the effects of BHT, both good and bad, occur at high doses, much higher than the amounts we ingest incidentally every day. However, the long-term effects of even the small doses that we use are poorly understood, and the wisdom of ingesting even these small amounts might well be questioned. There have been no human studies at these doses with BHT for herpes treatment or for safety. On the other hand, this chemical has passed the preliminaries of developing a new antiherpes drug—it works in the test tube and, at least in some investigators' hands, on the skin of animals. It was next tried on the skin of humans in a trial conducted by Dr. S. Spruance from the University of Utah. This double-blind, placebo-controlled trial failed to show any significant benefit. At this point, there is no precedent for humans to ingest BHT orally in these doses. Orally, it should be avoided until more information becomes available. Topically, it is not helpful.

L-lysine

L-lysine is a naturally occurring substance called an amino acid. Amino acids are the building blocks of all proteins. Proteins in the body are used to make the structure that holds us up and the molecular array that runs our metabolic processes. Our bodies have immense control over amino acids because we depend on them so much. We are constantly making and destroying amino acids and connecting them one to the other in order to maintain the exquisite balance just so.

In the 1960s, an effect of L-lysine against herpes simplex virus was noted in the test tube. It seems that changing the nutritional environment of herpes alters its capability to make its essential proteins. This amino acid balance can be critical, especially between two amino acids, lysine and arginine. These two amino acids work in somewhat opposite ways, in that lysine in excessive amounts damages the virus, while arginine in insufficient amounts has a similar effect. The lysine/arginine ratio is the important factor: a high ratio has a damaging effect on herpes simplex virus in culture. It is a giant leap to say that altering these chemicals in the diet will change the body's ability to combat clinical infection. In fact, it is not known whether this ratio can be changed in the body. There have been clinical trials with L-lysine, but they have never involved total dietary management, which is being suggested by a number of L-lysine advocates. The lysine work to date in humans is summarized below.

Dr. R. S. Griffith and his coworkers published an article in 1978 describing a multicenter trial of L-lysine for herpes infections.

Doses of 300 mg to 1,000 mg per day were used. A long-term beneficial effect was observed. However, this study had no control group. Many people with herpes swear by L-lysine, as popular trade magazines have attested. Without proper controls, however, placebo effects can be quite profound. In one study, 77 percent of 26 patients reported their oral herpes lesions to be markedly reduced in severity and duration by treatment with water! Ether, the test substance in that clinical trial, was shown to be no more effective than the water placebo. Back to L-lysine. If water works for 77 percent of people who think they are using a drug, then it would be wise to be very critical of studies that have no control group.

Two controlled trials of L-lysine have been performed in Denmark by Dr. N. Milman and his coworkers. First, L-lysine was used as treatment for recurrent oral herpes. The treatment was used as soon as a coming recurrence was sensed. It was tested on 251 recurrences. There was clearly no beneficial effect. Next, people with recurrent oral herpes took 1,000 mg daily, while the control group took starch powder tablets. After twelve weeks, the groups switched places. The drug had no effect on the number of recurrences, the rate of recurrences, the rate of healing of recurrences, or the symptoms of recurrences. Fourteen people had no recurrences at all during lysine treatment, whereas four people had no recurrences during starch treatment. This was considered to be of borderline significance.

In another study, from the Dermatology Branch at the National Institutes of Health in Bethesda, Maryland, Drs. J. DiGiovanna and H. Blank performed a randomized, double-blind, placebo-controlled trial of L-lysine taken for four to five months. The drug was given as 400 mg three times daily, and participants were advised not to take "excessive" amounts of seeds, nuts, or chocolate because of their arginine content. Their results were published in January 1984 in *Archives of Dermatology*. No substantial benefits of treatment were noted. The fact that only twenty patients were studied and follow-up during the treatment period was left mostly up to the patients themselves makes interpretation somewhat difficult. Nevertheless, all participants had a positive diagnosis at the time of entry, and no beneficial effects were seen.

In conclusion, it is not known whether the lysine/arginine ratio matters for herpes in humans. Dietary controls have only recently been part of the experimental design, and in this setting no benefits were noted. The average North American diet is much higher in lysine (meats and dairy products) than in arginine (legumes, whole grains, nuts). We do not know if altering the amino acid intake actually changes the nutrients available to the virus inside the cell. However, we are also in the dark concerning the safety of this regimen, because alterations of amino acids have undetermined effects on the body. Because amino acids are not called drugs, they are not controlled as drugs; as "natural" nutrients, they can be put into tablets and sold for consumption at any dosage.

2-deoxy-D-glucose (2-DG)

Glucose is simple sugar. Cells and viruses use simple sugar for a number of different processes. 2-DG is an analog of glucose. It is a look-alike as far as the metabolic system is concerned, so a cell needing a glucose molecule might grab and try to use a 2-DG molecule instead if one were around to grab. When viruses grab 2-DG, they seem to put the molecule into the virus envelope. This effectively stops herpes simplex growth by rendering the envelope useless. A lot of excitement was stirred up by a report in a June 1979 issue of the *Journal of the American Medical Association* stating that genital herpes infections could be effectively treated with this agent applied in a topical cream. The investigators claimed that this cream decreased the severity of the disease while it was being used and that it decreased the rate of subsequent recurrences. This study has come under intense criticism. In the study, the numbers of placebo patients was very small. In recurrent herpes episodes, the *average* number of days to healing of lesions was 12 after the placebo patients started using the cream, which occurred on average 4 days after the onset of symptoms. In other words, the healing time of the placebo group for a recurrence of herpes was more than two weeks—an extraordinary length of time. When compared to the treatment group's healing time of 6.8 days (plus the 4 days before using the cream) there was a great statistical difference. This means that drug recipients healed in 6.8 to 10.8 days, a standard and expected duration for an untreated recurrence.

The reasons for the very long placebo group healing time are unknown. No subsequent studies in humans with this drug have been published. This drug has been extensively tested against genital herpes in guinea pigs and mice. No positive effects were seen; it did not inhibit the development of sores, nor did it inhibit the quantity of virus present. It has been reported to be useful in rabbit eye infections with herpes simplex, although these effects are not impressive when compared to those of other antiviral agents.

For now, 2-DG is on the back burner. This compound is not available for the treatment of genital herpes or for other use.

Contraceptive foam

Nonoxynol-9 is a *surfactant*, a surface-active substance. It acts very similarly to soap. In the test tube, this agent, like soap, effectively inactivates herpes simplex virus. It was reported in early uncontrolled observations to be effective in the therapy of genital herpes infection. When tested in a placebo-controlled trial, however, nonoxynol-9 was not beneficial. Herpes lesions in recipients of this drug healed more slowly than those in the placebo group. One company is, however, selling this agent as a topical treatment for recurrent herpes. More promising data have come from using nonoxynol-9 in combination with topical interferon. Nonoxynol-9 is also a very important preventive tool, when used properly, in combination with a condom. As a preventive tool, nonoxynol-9 is safe and shows demonstrable antiviral effects in the test tube. It is capable of preventing transmission of herpes simplex virus in mice. Too much use of nonoxynol-9 can actually induce chafing and ulceration of the vaginal wall, however, so use should probably be limited to once or twice daily as a maximum. (See chapter 12 for further information.)

Lithium

Lithium is effective against herpes in the test tube. It inactivates herpes simplex at a concentration of 30 to 60 milliequivalents. This is 20 to 60 times the levels considered appropriate for treating humans for manic-depressive illness (the only clinical setting where lithium should be used).

Very few people with herpes have been reportedly helped (for herpes) by lithium. Furthermore, lithium has very important and potentially dangerous side effects. Lithium is dangerous except under the rigid control of experts administering it. It should not be used for herpes except as part of a carefully controlled clinical trial.

Zinc

Zinc is also capable of inhibiting herpes simplex virus in the test tube. It is a common component of various skin creams. Zinc has been tried as a cream combined with ultrasound treatment and has also been given by mouth. Neither of these settings, although reported in the literature, was set up as a trial with placebo controls, randomization, etc. Conclusions cannot be drawn.

Dimethyl sulfoxide (DMSO)

This organic solvent rapidly penetrates skin. It is so effective at penetrating skin that some recipients have been able to taste it in the mouth within seconds of applying it to the skin surface. DMSO is also very effective at carrying antiviral agents with it. Thus, it has been thought that mixing a good drug in DMSO may make it penetrate better and therefore work better. In the case of topical acyclovir, DMSO does markedly enhance drug penetration through the skin of guinea pigs. DMSO has been tried clinically in the case of idoxuridine. Early reports suggested that a combination of idoxuridine with DMSO might be an effective herpes treatment. In an exhaustive study published in the *Journal of the American Medical Association* in August 1982, however, Drs. Silvestri, Corey, and Holmes found that idoxuridine in DMSO had no clinical effect on primary or recurrent herpes. People receiving the treatment complained of burning and allergy. One person developed local cancer at the site of drug application. In a study of idoxuridine in DMSO used for herpes labialis (cold sores), Dr. S. L. Spruance and colleagues reported in the *Journal of Infectious Diseases* that the combination appeared to offer some minor benefits. Using DMSO as a penetration enhancer makes a lot of theoretical sense. Perhaps a different penetration enhancer with the right topical drug will allow topical antivirals to be used more effectively in the future; penetration enhancers are being considered with some drugs. DMSO is not currently indicated for the treatment of herpes, either alone or in combination with an antiviral agent.

Adenosine monophosphate (AMP)

In 1979, Drs. S. H. Sklar and E. Buimovici-Klein reported that adenosine-5'-monophosphate (AMP) was effective in the treatment of patients with recurrent oral herpes. AMP was given by nine to twelve intramuscular injections on alternate days. The authors claimed from this uncontrolled study that pain and discomfort were ameliorated quickly. AMP is a natural cellular compound. Side effects (which were not extensively looked for) were not seen. It has been suggested that this agent might stabilize membranes in the nervous system and thus prevent reactivation. Studies of recurring herpes simplex infection in mice have suggested that AMP might be able to prevent recurrences under certain experimental conditions. Although the animal results were interesting, these studies were also not placebo-controlled, and thus the results are difficult to interpret.

In the March 8, 1985, issue of the *Journal of the American Medical Association*, Drs. Sklar, Blue, Alexander, and Bodian demonstrated a useful effect on the treatment of herpes zoster infections (shingles). Their trial was double-blind, randomized, and placebo-controlled. Their numbers were small (thirty-two volunteers in total). The drug was put into gel and injected intramuscularly three times per week. Further clinical trials will be necessary.

Other treatments

The following agents have not been reported as proven effective against herpes in a clinical trial using placebos and controls. Thus, their usefulness is unknown. Some have received anecdotal treatment in the scientific literature. In other words, they may have been suggested as possibly effective, but the numbers or the design of the experiment were not possible to evaluate. These agents include acidophilus, acupuncture, aloe vera, antibiotics, aspirin, heat, ice, ginseng, herbal mixtures, homeopathic treatment, hypnosis, laser therapy, ozone therapy, povidone-iodine (Betadine), red algae extract, transcendental meditation, vitamin B complex, vitamin B12, vitamin C, and vitamin E.

The following compounds have been tested in scientific studies and have been shown to be ineffective. The ones marked with an asterisk (*) are also considered worse than using nothing, either because they may prolong lesions or complications, or because of real or potential harmful effects or local discomfort upon application:

- alcohol applied to the sores
- Bacille Calmette-Guerin (BCG) vaccine*
- chloroform* applied to the sores
- DMSO* (Rimso-50, dimethyl sulfoxide) applied to the sores
- ether* applied to the sores
- idoxuridine (IDU, Stoxil, Herplex-D) applied to the sores
- levamisole*
- nonoxynol-9* applied to the sores
- ointments or creams not containing a specific antiherpes drug (including cortisone, antibiotics, etc.)*
- oral polio vaccine
- photodynamic inactivation (light and red dye treatments)*
- smallpox vaccine*
- topical adenine arabinoside (Vira-A, ara-A)

12
Condoms
and Safer Sex

...until Love Story is remade with moving episodes of con-
dom-related sex play, the rubber sheath will continue to be
associated with casual sex and fear of disease. Failure to
glamourise the condom may have serious consequences.

—GERMAINE GREER

Sex and Destiny:
The Politics of Human Fertility

What is a condom exactly?

The condom is a penis sheath, usually made out of latex rubber or
a membrane from sheep intestine. Historians suggest that Gabriele
Fallopio was the first to use a linen sheath as protection from
syphilis. England's King Charles II was apparently the first user of
the membrane prophylactic. Early penis covers were made from
the gastrointestinal tracts of sheep or other animals. While its precise origins are not certain, many believe that Charles's physician,
Dr. Condom, designed the device to prevent the birth of unwanted
children of his king's mistresses. Casanova went on to describe
condom use in great detail during the eighteenth century. High
cost limited condom use at that time to the upper classes of
Europe. By the middle of the nineteenth century, however, the
process of vulcanization of rubber allowed the price of condoms
to drop considerably. During the 1930s, more than 300 million latex
condoms were sold annually in the United States. Along came the
birth control pill, the intrauterine device, and the diaphragm, and
the condom business suffered. Along came genital herpes, and the
condom business continued to suffer. Along came AIDS, and the
condom business has never been the same. Latex condoms may
literally be one of the keys to world survival.

Who should be using condoms?

The condom is a birth control device that, when properly used, also prevents transmission of most sexually transmitted diseases. Let us first consider the theoretical ideal. If every individual used condoms along with the spermicidal agent nonoxynol-9 each time he or she had sexual intercourse until such time as both partners agreed to enter a permanent, monogamous relationship, AIDS and most other sexually transmitted diseases would begin to vanish from the earth. That is how effective these things are, if used correctly. Concerning genital herpes, later in this chapter I advise that condoms be used only during the inactive phases of infection. From a *statistical* point of view, of course, they would reduce transmission even when used in the active phases. From the *individual's* point of view, however, neither protected nor unprotected sexual contact with the affected area of skin is advised during the active phases of herpes. Condoms are recommended for nearly everyone, regardless of whether you or your partner have genital herpes. If one partner does have genital herpes the condom, properly used, may add a new and very attractive element to the relationship— peace of mind.

Forget any previous prejudices against condoms. If you've never tried them before, now is the time. If you've tried them before and didn't like the experience, it is time to try again. The market is now flooded with condoms in all shapes, sizes, colors, and flavors. Some condoms are extra tight at the base to restrict leakage after ejaculation and possibly prolong the time before ejaculation. Some are ribbed to increase pleasure. They are easy to obtain in drug stores, convenience stores, and even by mail order. No prescription is required. They can be used only when needed, unlike pills and devices that require advance planning. Condoms require no premeditation, although they do have to be carried just in case. Whether you are male or female, carrying condoms is thoughtful and appropriate and not a sign of being after only one thing; people who keep condoms with them are responsible people who care about their own health and the health of their partners. Furthermore, people committed to making condoms work for them will find little to diminish the pleasure of sex. They are easy to use and can actually be made a part of the sexual experience, possibly even enhancing it.

Condoms work. They prevent disease and pregnancy. Previously reported failure rates of up to 10 percent are highly inflated. Most of these numbers include people who used condoms improperly or who sometimes forgot to use them at all. The fact that in a recent study of physicians using condoms for birth control no pregnancies occurred suggests that misuse is a more likely cause of failure than the device itself. Properly used, the condom prevents pregnancy a bit better than the intrauterine device and the diaphragm and about the same as the birth control pill. Using the right condom in the right way is the only trick.

Will condoms prevent the transmission of infections?

Latex condoms properly tested by the manufacturer (choose products from reputable companies) will not allow the passage of infectious agents of any kind—for example, HIV (the virus that causes AIDS), herpes simplex virus, hepatitis B virus, human papillomavirus (the cause of genital warts), cytomegalovirus, Chlamydia, gonorrhea, and syphilis. The same may not be true for some "natural" condoms made from the intestines of animals. These membranes are more variable in their pore sizes and, while perfectly good at preventing pregnancy, they may not be as good at preventing disease. Further scientific work needs to be done to sort out the subtle differences between one type and another. For now, in trying to prevent transmission of herpes, choose condoms made from latex rubber. In case of allergy to latex, plastic condoms are now available.

In my opinion, it is preferable to use condoms containing the spermicidal agent nonoxynol-9. This safe, soaplike substance, which kills sperm, also kills the herpes virus in the test tube and prevents transmission of genital herpes in mice. It is even being tested, in combination with other drugs, as a possible antiviral treatment. One study showed that even if a condom broke, the AIDS virus (HIV) was inactivated two-thirds of the time by nonoxynol-9 when it was present in the tip of the condom. Nonoxynol-9 can also be used by the woman or recipient male partner as a contraceptive foam, serving to aid lubrication and further prevent disease transmission.

Unfortunately, nonoxynol-9 can also be irritating for some people. Irritation potential increases with repeated uses in short periods of time. Some studies have shown microulceration of the genital skin with frequent use. Such irritation could have the effect of making virus entry easier. Thus, nonoxynol-9's use has become controversial. It is generally a good product and a good idea unless it irritates your skin or you use it very frequently.

Several new spermicides and topical antiviral agents are being studied in animals to determine if there might be a better product that can do more to prevent virus transmission. Never use oil-based products like Vaseline or mineral oil to lubricate latex condoms, as they dissolve them and make holes. Several proven water-based lubricants are available that are specifically designed for use with condoms. Some have nonoxynol-9 added and others do not. Some are flavored; others are not. If you are not completely certain whether a particular lubricant should be used with condoms, do not use it.

For birth control, condoms are effective but not ideal. Ideal protection from pregnancy and disease transmission is obtained by combining condoms and safer sex practices as outlined below with a second method of birth control—for example, the birth control pill. The birth control pill provides no protection against herpes, AIDS, or any other sexually transmitted disease, however.

What about female condoms?

Female condoms are now available. The female condom is inserted by the female partner before contact and serves as a protective lining of the female genital tract. The area of protection is much wider, as the condom covers a much more extensive mucosal and skin surface than the male version. The material is a bit different, also. It is a good idea, theoretically, although it might take some getting used to for some couples. From the herpes point of view, the female condom is theoretically even more attractive, since it covers the vulvar surface, where herpes might still have access from an uncovered portion of the man's genitals. I am not aware of any specific data regarding herpes and the female condom. It is a new and under-used resource, so far. It might be very interesting to give it a try, if you wish.

Are there any special precautions to take?

Yes. Nothing replaces common sense. Remember these points:

1. Condoms cover the penis—the shaft and the tip (glans). They do not cover the base of the shaft, the scrotum, or the pubic hair areas, which are commonly contacted during intercourse. It is unwise to have genital sexual contact during the active phases of infection, whether you elect to use a condom or not and whether the affected area of skin is covered by the condom or not.

2. Furthermore, although using a condom during the inactive phases of infection prevents a significant proportion of herpes transmission, prevention is not *guaranteed*. In the unlikely event of asymptomatic shedding in vaginal secretions, if the nonoxynol-9 does not inactivate the virus, and if secretions remain at the base of the penis for a prolonged period after intercourse, it is still *possible* to transmit herpes.

3. Condoms may break because of manufacturing defects but tests performed by the major manufacturers make this extremely unlikely. Look for the words "electronically tested" on the package. Causes of breakage unrelated to manufacturing problems are much more common and easy to avoid. They include inadequate lubrication (the most common cause), use of the wrong lubrication which weakens the device (see below), use of outdated condoms, or ones that have been left in the heat or sun or allowed to dry out because of a tear in the package. In addition, condoms may be torn accidentally with teeth, fingernails, or jewelry.

Are there some simple guidelines to follow?

Dr. Robert Hatcher is a professor of gynecology and obstetrics at Emory University School of Medicine. His book, *Contraceptive Technology 1986/1987*, is recommended for further information.

He offers "rules" of "condom sense." I have liberally added to and edited his rules for this book, since the transmission of genital herpes is unique among the sexually transmitted infections. Selected advice gleaned from work by Ansell Inc., Dotham, Alabama, and the Départements de Santé Communautaire du Québec is also incorporated into my version of these rules:

1. If you elect to use condoms for preventing virus transmission, use quality latex condoms. If you are unsure about products, ask the pharmacist or your physician which brands are preferred. Use a condom every single time you have intercourse. There should be no exceptions.

2. Put the condom on as soon as complete erection occurs. Unprotected contact with any orifice—vagina, mouth, or rectum—is the same as not using a condom at all as regards transmission. In other words, it is not enough to put the condom on after you have begun having intercourse but before ejaculation. If you want to protect yourself and your partner against all sexually transmitted infections, then you will want to avoid unprotected contact altogether, whether this is genital-genital, genital-oral, oral-anal, or whatever. Virtually all sexually transmitted infections other than genital herpes are not periodic. Transmission could occur during any sexual contact.

3. If your main reason for using condoms is to prevent asymptomatic transmission of genital herpes, then refer also to chapter 5 on transmission, which discusses these issues in detail. Since genital herpes is periodic, with active and inactive phases, short-term unprotected contact (e.g., oral-genital) is unlikely to result in transmission during inactive phases of infection. However, the growing information on the risk of asymptomatic shedding and asymptomatic transmission of herpes strongly requires that you adopt safer sexual practices during inactive (asymptomatic) phases of infection. Your choice about unprotected oral-genital contact, and so on, should be based on various factors and should be made mutually with your partner. If you and your partner have decided to use condoms to prevent asymptomatic transmission of genital herpes, then mixing pro-

tected genital sexual contact with unprotected oral-genital contact is inconsistent. It is possible, by the way, to add barrier latex protection to oral-genital contact through the use of latex sheets. You can cut a regular latex condom into a square sheet and use it that way. Others use latex dental dams or microwaveable plastic wrap.

4. Squeeze any air out of the tip of the condom by holding the tip between the fingers of one hand as you put it on. Air bubbles tend to interfere with sensation and may cause breakage. Be careful of sharp corners on your fingernails while handling the condom, since they could tear the rubber.

5. Place the condom on the penis *only after* complete erection occurs, but *before any* contact between penis and partner. Roll the condom's rim all the way to the base of the penis before the penis touches the partner. Do not unroll the condom before putting it on.

6. If the condom lacks a reservoir tip, leave a small empty space (about half an inch) at the tip to catch semen. Better yet, use a condom with a built-in reservoir tip. (Remember to keep the air out of the reservoir tip by squeezing it as you put it on.)

7. For lubrication, do not use petroleum jelly (for example, Vaseline), mineral oil, vegetable shortening or oil, or any other oil-based lubricant, because they may deteriorate the latex. Saliva is also *not* an appropriate lubricant. Sufficient lubrication is essential to prevent the condom from tearing. Most people choose to use prelubricated condoms. If further lubrication is required, use water, or water-based lubricants made especially for this purpose (for example, KY Jelly), or spermicidal jelly or spermicidal foam. You can purchase these with or without nonoxynol-9. Maximum protection generally supports using nonoxynol-9, as part of the condom lubricant, as a component of foam, jelly, or cream, or (best choice) as a component of both. However, there is some controversy about this.

8. After intercourse, the partner wearing the condom should hold onto the rim of the condom as the penis is withdrawn, being careful not to spill any of its contents. Withdraw the penis from

the partner soon after ejaculation, because as the erection is lost, the condom may slip off and allow semen to escape.

9. Do not use a condom more than once. Condoms are not washable or reusable. Dispose of the condom safely so that no one (a child, for example) has access to it.

10. Store unused condoms in a cool, dry place. Do not keep them in a wallet, a glove compartment, a dashboard, or any other hot place for a long time, because heat can deteriorate the latex. Condoms keep well in a purse or a shirt/jacket pocket.

11. Most companies now put expiry dates on condom boxes. Check for the date, and make sure it is appropriate. If no date is given, keep in mind that condoms kept in their foil package protected from light and heat will stay fresh for about five years.

12. It is a good idea to open a condom package on your own before you begin using condoms during sexual encounters. Check to see what a condom looks like and feels like and how it unrolls, etc. But use a spare for this. Do not plan to use this test condom as the real thing later on, since testing it will damage it.

13. The standard condom may not resist breakage during anal sex. New brands made of a thicker latex are beginning to appear on the market for this purpose and are preferred. These brands usually require a lot of lubrication.

What does the term "safer sex" really mean?

Recently, we have been inundated with material suggesting the practice of "safer sex" to prevent the transmission of all sexually transmitted diseases. The AIDS epidemic, of course, is the main stimulus behind this effort. Such an approach should be supported vigorously in order to control infection. The term "safe sex," rather than "safer sex," would be misleading. If a condom is used incorrectly or left in the drawer, barrier contraception provides no benefit. The techniques of safer sex definitely enhance—indeed, *markedly* enhance—the safety of sex in general. They make sex *safer*. They do *not* make sex 100 percent safe. Condoms prevent the transmission of most diseases that might otherwise be transmitted by penile-vaginal or penile-anal or penile-oral sex. Since condoms cover the penis effectively when used properly, they make most sexual contact a lot safer. Additional safer sex methods that are becoming available include female condoms, for use by women during genital sexual intercourse, and latex barriers (also called "dental dams") for use in oral sexual contact. Condoms can also be carefully cut with scissors and reshaped for use in oral sex. These methods effectively reduce risks.

Combining safer sex practices and a reduction in the number of sexual partners further reduces the risk of sexually transmitted diseases. Being selective does not mean that you should avoid people who are honest enough to tell you that they have genital herpes. Being selective does not mean that you are safe from infection if you feel that you are in love. That is certainly a good start in building a relationship, but other factors should be borne in mind when trying to prevent infection. Many of my patients are shocked to learn that they have acquired genital herpes, because they feel they have "always been very careful." Usually this means that they have known someone well and trusted them before having a sexual relationship, or that they have limited their partners to others they thought were "clean." As I have stated in many places in this book, genital herpes affects "good people," "clean people," and "trustworthy people." Only special medical tests can reveal who has herpes and who does not. Sexually transmitted diseases very often cause no obvious symptoms, and they do not limit themselves to people who are not lovable. Therefore, if your partner is in a high risk group for sexually transmitted infections other than AIDS (i.e., if their previous sexual partners have been very high in number or occasionally anonymous or casual), then examination for sexually transmitted infection by a competent health care provider is indicated, preferably before having sex, and especially before having unprotected sex. If any genital symptoms are present, regardless of how mild they are, then the same rules should apply. Such examinations are easy to obtain. A clean bill of health on one examination does not rule out genital herpes. However, it can rule out nearly everything else, if done properly. Genital herpes can only be ruled out with a special blood test called the Western blot. This is a simple blood test but needs to be performed in a special laboratory. It is discussed at length in chapter 4. Other tests for herpes are also discussed in that chapter.

If your partner is in a risk group for AIDS, it is easy, anonymous, and usually free of charge for your partner to find out if he or she is infected with HIV. High risk groups include people with the following:

- A history of unprotected male homosexual or bisexual contact since 1976.

- A history of intravenous drug use since 1976.

- A history of receiving unscreened blood products, including transfusions or hemophilia factors, or organ transplants since 1976. Most exposure via these routes has now ceased because of donor screening, which began in March/April of 1985.

- Recipient of artificial insemination between 1976 and 1985.

- A history of being exposed to needles used for intravenous applications in humans, e.g. hospital workers with specific, unprotected high-level exposure to blood products.

- A history of sexual contact with a prostitute since 1976.

- A history of sexual contact with a native of one of many African countries, Haiti, and Southeast Asia. The list of places where AIDS is becoming commonplace is rapidly increasing, especially in the poorest parts of the Third World.

- A history of being a sexual partner of anyone in a high-risk group listed above.

- A history of many heterosexual relationships since 1976 and especially in the past few years.

Find out before you have sexual contact. That is safe. Not finding out and having sex with a condom is safer than not using a condom. In fact, the condom method is safer by a factor of ten times or more, based on transmission studies with AIDS in long-term relationships. Even so, if you seek sex that is 100 percent safe, you are advised to delay sex until you know whether your partner carries HIV. Furthermore, one AIDS test alone is only adequate if the reason for the partner's high risk has ceased to exist. If the partner's possible exposure to HIV is ongoing, one test will not provide reassurance of safety. Before you or your partner have an AIDS test or interpret the results of an AIDS test, you should be offered thorough counseling about the issues.

If herpes is your only concern regarding transmission, then even without using condoms, couples often avoid transmission. Yet, data are clear that avoiding sex just at times of symptoms, and not using safer sex practices poses a very real risk of herpes transmission to an uninfected partner. The risks of asymptomatic shedding are discussed in detail in chapter 5. Using condoms properly during inactive phases offers added protection and makes transmission much less likely than without protection. One study from UCLA found asymptomatic genital herpes transmission between partners only in couples who did not routinely practice safer sex. Precise statistics are not available on asymptomatic transmission risks with the use of safer sex precautions.

Permissions

Appendix 1:
Resources

The following is a list of organizations and publications in the U.S. or Canada that provide information on herpes. Several herpes telephone lines are now available. You will also want to get involved with a good health care professional who can provide proper diagnosis, treatment and counseling.

U.S. hotline services include:

Herpes Advice Centers Hotline: 1-888-ADVICE-8
Trained counselors will answer questions about herpes. Educational materials can be ordered and are sent through the mail in privacy envelopes.

National Herpes Hotline: (919) 361-8488
To order an information packet, call 1-800-230-6039.

Operated by the Herpes Resource Center, a program of the American Social Health Association (ASHA). The center publishes free written information about herpes which they will mail to you in a privacy envelope via the toll-free lines. Trained counselors are available to answer questions about herpes through the long distance access number.

Sexually Transmitted Disease Information and Referral Center Hotline: 1-800-653-HEALTH.
Also sponsored by the American Social Health Association, this hotline uses recorded information about sexually transmitted diseases. Herpes publications can be faxed to you.

CDC National STD Hotline: 1-800-227-8922
Operated by the U.S. Centers for Disease Control and Prevention and ASHA. Callers can request free, written information about herpes or other sexually transmitted diseases. Hotline operators can also refer you to a public health

clinic in your area for diagnosis and treatment of herpes or other sexually transmitted diseases.

Publications available through the ASHA (prices may have changed since the publication of this book):

The Helper

A quarterly newsletter, published by the ASHA, discusses herpes issues and the latest research. Ordered through the National Herpes Hotline or write ASHA, Department T, PO Box 13827, Research Triangle Park, NC 27709. A year's subscription is $25.00.

Sexual Health: The Magazine for Sexual Well-Being

A bimonthly consumer magazine that covers a wide range of topics. Subscriptions are $20.00 per year. 1-888-ADVICE-8.

Managing Herpes: How to Live and Love with a Chronic STD.

A 224-page guide to emotional and medical issues, published by ASHA. $17.95.

Understanding Herpes

A 20-page information booklet about herpes which is packaged with two brochures: "Telling Your Partner", and "When Your Partner Has Herpes." $7.00.

Living with Herpes...The Facts and the Feelings

An 18-minute video available from ASHA. $19.95.

SmithKline Beecham provides an educational website about genital herpes at http://www.cafeherpe.com. They offer information about viruses, the physical and emotional aspects of genital herpes, and where to find genital herpes resources and support centers. You can also reach the Viridae website at http://www.viridae.com. We provide information about our research services as well as an extensive information packet which summarizes much of what is contained in this book.

APPENDIX 2:

Additional Reading

The following list of books and articles on the subject of herpes is recommended for those who wish to read more. This list is not intended to be a complete bibliography or reference section for this book. You will need to visit a medical library for access to all of these articles except those with an asterisk (*). They are selected for inclusion in this section because they are, more or less, readable by a nonprofessional.

To find a medical library, you may call your local medical society and ask. Often the society or local hospital will have their own. A trip to a university with a medical school is occasionally necessary. Call locally first, because often a local small library will be able to obtain a copy of an article on a specific subject by interlibrary loan.

GENERAL TOPICS: HERPES SIMPLEX VIRUS

Kaplan A.S., ed. *The Herpes Viruses.* New York: Academic Press, 1973.

Nahmias A.J.; Dowdle, W.R.; and Schinazi, R.F., eds. *The Human Herpes Viruses: An Interdisciplinary Perspective.* New York: Elsevier North Holland, 1981.

Nahmias A.J., and Roizman, B. "Infection with herpes simplex viruses 1 and 2." *New England Journal of Medicine* 289 (1973): 667-674, 719-725, 781-789.

Richman D.D., Whitley R.J., Hayden F.G. *Clinical Virology.* City: Churchill Livingstone, 1996.

Wyatt L.S., and Frenkel N. "Human herpesvirus 7 is a constitutive inhabitant of adult human saliva." *Journal of Virology* 66 (1992): 3206-3209.

GENITAL HERPES INFECTION

Adams H.G., et al. "Genital herpetic infection in men and women: clinical course and effect of topical application of adenine arabinoside." *The Journal of Infectious Diseases* 133 Supplement (1976): A151-A159.

Ashley R.L., et al. "Comparison of Western blot (immunoblot) and glyco-protein G-specific immunodot enzyme assay for assay for detecting anti-bodies to herpes simplex virus types 1 and 2 in human sera." *Journal of Clinical Microbiology* 26 (1988): 662-667.

Ashley R.L., et al. "Inability of enzyme immunoassays to discriminate between infections with herpes simplex virus types 1 and 2." *Annals of Internal Medicine* 115 (1991): 520-526.

Barton S.E., et al. "Screening to detect asymptomatic shedding of herpes simplex virus (HSV) in women with recurrent genital HSV infection." *Genitourinary Medicine* 62 (1986): 181-185.

Bernstein D.I., et al. "Serologic analysis of first-episode nonprimary genital herpes simplex virus Infection: presence of type 2 antibody in acute serum samples." *The American Journal of Medicine* 77 (1984): 1055-1060.

Brock BV, et al. "Frequency of asymptomatic shedding of herpes simplex virus in women with genital herpes." *The Journal of The American Medical Association* 263 (1990): 418-420.

Brown Z.A., et al. "Clinical and virologic course of herpes simplex genital-is." *Western Journal of Medicine* 130 (1979): 414-421.

Corey L. "The diagnosis and treatment of genital herpes." *Journal of the American Medical Association* 248 (1982): 1041-1049.

Corey L., et al. "Genital herpes simplex infections: clinical manifestations, course, and complications." *Annals of Internal Medicine* 98 (1983): 958-972.

Dalessio J., and Ashley R. "Highly sensitive enhanced chemiluminescence immunodetection method for herpes simplex virus type 2 Western immunoblot." *Journal of Clinical Microbiology* 30(1992): 1005-1007.

Guinan M.E., et al. "The course of untreated recurrent genital herpes sim-plex infection in 27 women." *New England Journal of Medicine* 304 (1981): 759-763.

Hardy DA, et al. "Use of polymerase chain reaction for successful identifi-cation of asymptomatic genital infection with herpes simplex virus in pregnant women at delivery." *Journal of Infectious Diseases* 162 (1990): 1031-1035.

Harger J.H., et al. "Changes in the frequency of genital herpes simplex recurrences as a function of time." *Obstetrics and Gynecology* 67 (1986): 637-642.

Ho D.W., et al. "Indirect ELISA for the detection of HSV-2 specific IgG and IgM antibodies with glycoprotein G (gG-2)." *Journal of Virological Methods* 36 (1992): 249-264.

Koelle D.M. "Asymptomatic reactivation of herpes simplex virus in women after the first episode of genital herpes." *Annals of Internal Medicine* 116 (1992): 433-437.

Koutsky L.A., et al. "Underdiagnosis of genital herpes by current clinical and viral-isolation procedures." *New England Journal of Medicine* 326 (1992): 1533-1539.

Lafferty W.E., et al. "Recurrences after oral and genital herpes simplex virus infection: influence of site infection and viral type." *New England Journal of Medicine* 316 (1987): 1444-1449.

Langenberg A., et al. "Development of clinically recognizable genital lesions among women previously identified as having 'asymptomatic' herpes simplex virus type 2 infection." *Annals of Internal Medicine* 110 (1989): 882-887.

Mertz G.J., et al. "Frequency of acquisition of first-episode genital infection with herpes simplex virus from symptomatic and asymptomatic source contacts." *Sexually Transmitted Diseases.* 12 (1985): 33-39.

Mertz G.J., et al. "Risk factors for the sexual transmission of genital herpes." *Annals of Internal Medicine* 116 (1992): 197-202.

Rooney J.F., et al. "Acquisition of genital herpes from an asymptomatic sexual partner." *New England Journal of Medicine* 314 (1986): 1561-1564.

Sacks S.L. "Frequency and duration of patient-observed recurrent genital herpes simplex virus infection: characterization of the nonlesional prodrome." *Journal of Infectious Diseases* 150 (1984): 873-877.

Sacks S.L., and Koss, M. "The emotional and physical consequences of genital herpes simplex virus infection." Programs and Abstracts of the 26th Interscience Conference on Antimicrobial Agents and Chemotherapy. Washington: *American Society for Microbiology,* 1986.

Sacks S.L., et al. "Clinical course of recurrent genital herpes and treatment with foscarnet cream: results of a Canadian multicenter trial." *Journal of Infectious Diseases* 155 (1987): 178-186.

Stenzel-Poore M.P., et al. "Herpes simplex virus shedding in genital secretions." *Sexually Transmitted Diseases* 14 (1987): 17-22.

Straus S.E., et al. "Effect of oral acyclovir treatment on symptomatic and asymptomatic virus shedding in recurrent genital herpes." *Sexually Transmitted Diseases.* 16 (1989): 107-113.

Vontver L.A., et al. "Clinical course and diagnosis of genital herpes simplex virus infection and evaluation of topical surfactant therapy." *American Journal of Obstetrics and Gynecology* (1979): 548-554.

HERPES OF THE NEWBORN

Arvin A.M., and Prober, C.G. "Herpes simplex virus infections: the genital tract and the newborn." *Pediatric Reviews* 13(1992): 107-112.

Bradley J.S., et al. "Neutralization of herpes simplex virus by antibody in amniotic fluid." *Obstetrics and Gynecology* 60 (1982): 318-321.

Brown Z.A., et al. "Effects on infants of a first episode of genital herpes during pregnancy." *New England Journal of Medicine* 317 (1987): 1246-1251.

Brown Z.A., et al. "Neonatal herpes simplex virus infection in relation to asymptomatic maternal infection at the time of labor." *New England Journal of Medicine* 324 (1991): 1247-1252.

Committee on Fetus and Newborn. Committee on Infectious Diseases. "Perinatal herpes simplex virus infections." *Pediatrics* 66 (1980): 147-149.

Frenkel L.M., et al. "Clinical reactivation of herpes simplex virus type-2 infection in seropositive pregnant women with no history of genital herpes." *Annals of Internal Medicine* 118 (1993): 414-418.

Haddad J., et al. "Oral acyclovir and recurrent genital herpes during late pregnancy." *Obstetrics & Gynecology* 82 (1993): 102-104.

Harger J.H., et al. "Characteristics and management of pregnancy in women with genital herpes simplex virus infection." *American Journal of Obstetrics and Gynecology* (1983): 784-791.

Honig P.J., et al. "Congenital herpes simplex virus infections." *Archives of Dermatology* 115 (1979): 1329-1333.

Kibrick S. "Herpes simplex infection at term: what to do with mother, newborn and nursery personnel." *Journal of the American Medical Association* 243 (1980): 157-160.

Kulhanjian J.A., et al. "Identification of women at unsuspected risk of primary infection with herpes simplex virus type 2 during pregnancy." *New England Journal of Medicine* 326 (1992): 916-920.

Nahmias A.J., Keyserling, H.L., and Kerrick, G.M. "Herpes Simplex." *Infectious Diseases of the Fetus and Newborn Infant.* Edited by J.S. Remington and J.O. Klein. Philadelphia: W.B. Saunders, 1983.

Prober C.G., et al. "The management of pregnancies complicated by genital infections with herpes simplex virus." *Clinical Infectious Diseases,* 15 (1992): 1031-1038.

Randolph A.G., et al. "Cesarean delivery for women presenting with genital herpes lesions. efficacy, risks, and costs." *Journal of The American Medical Association* 270 (1993): 77-82.

Vontver L.A., et al. "Recurrent genital herpes simplex virus infection in pregnancy: infant outcome and frequency of asymptomatic recurrences." *American Journal of Obstetrics and Gynecology* 143 (1982): 75-81.

Whitley R.J., et al. "Changing presentation of HSV infection in neonates." *Journal of Infectious Diseases* 158 (1988): 109-116.

Yeager A.S., et al. "Relationship of antibody to outcome in neonatal herpes simplex virus infections." *Infection and Immunity* 29 (1980): 532-538

HERPES AND CANCER

Barnett R., and Fox R. A Feminist Approach To Pap Tests. Available for postage from the *Vancouver Women's Health Collective,* 1501 West Broadway, Vancouver, B.C. V6J 1W6. (604) 736-4234*

Kaufman R.H., et al. "Herpes virus-induced antigens in squamous cell carcinoma in situ of the vulva." *New England Journal of Medicine* 305 (1981): 483-488.

Nahmias A.J., and Sawanabori S. "The genital herpes-cervical cancer hypothesis—10 years later." *Progress in Experimental Tumor Research 21* (1978): 117-139.

Rawls W.E., et al. "An analysis of seroepidemiological studies of herpes virus type 2 and carcinoma of the cervix." *Cancer Research* 33 (1973): 1477-1482.

Schachter J. "Sexually transmitted infections and cervical atypia." *Sexually Transmitted Diseases* 8 (1981): 353-356.

Bergeron C.R., et al. "Human papillomavirus associated with cervical intraepithelial neoplasia." *American Journal of Surgical Pathology* 16 (1992): 641-649.

Kruman R.J. "Basaloid and warty carcinomas of the vulva." *American Journal of Surgical Pathology* 17 (1993): 133-145.

HERPES AND PSYCHOLOGY

Bok S. *Lying: Moral Choice in Public and Private Life.* New York: Pantheon Books, 1978.

Bok S. *Secrets: On the Ethics of Concealment and Revelation.* New York: Pantheon Books, 1983.

Catotti D.N., et al. "Herpes revisited: still a cause of concern." *Sexually Transmitted Diseases,* 20 (1993): 77-80.

Keller M.L. et al. "Perceived stressors and coping responses in persons with recurrent genital herpes." *Research in Nursing and Health* 14 (1991): 421-430.

Kinghorn G.R. "Addressing the psychosocial needs of genital herpes sufferers [letter]." *Genitourinary Medicine* 68 (1992): 424

Kubler-Ross E. *On Death and Dying.* New York: MacMillan, 1969.*

Russell J.M., et al. "Management of genital herpes by genitourinary physicians: does experience or doctor's gender influence clinical management?" *Genitourinary Medicine,* 69 (1993): 115-118.

Selye H. *Stress Without Distress.* Signet Books: New York, 1975.*

NONGENITAL HERPES

Bader C., et al. "The natural history of recurrent facial-oral infection with herpes simplex virus." *Journal of Infectious Diseases* 138 (1978): 897-905.

Cavanagh H.D. "Herpetic ocular disease: therapy of persistent epithelial defects." *International Ophthalmology Clinics* 15 (1975): 67-88.

Detjen P.F., et al. "Herpes simplex virus associated with recurrent Stevens-Johnson syndrome: a management strategy." *Archives of Internal Medicine* 152 (1992): 1513-1516.

Gill M.J., et al. "Herpes simplex virus infection of the hand: a profile of 79 cases." *The American Journal of Medicine 84* (1988): 89-93.

Wassilew S.W. "Treatment of herpes simplex of the skin: critical evaluation of antiherpetic drugs with reference to relative potency on the eye." *Advances in Ophthalmology* 38 (1979): 125-133.

Whitley R.J., et al. "Adenine arabinoside therapy of biopsy-proved herpes simplex encephalitis: National Institute of Allergy and Infectious Diseases Collaborative Antiviral Study." *New England Journal of Medicine* 297 (1977): 289-294.

Whitley R.J., and Schlitt M. "Encephalitis caused by herpesviruses, including B virus." In: Scheld W.M., Whitley, R.J., and Durack D.T. (eds.) Infections of the Central Nervous System, New York, *Raven Press,* 1991, pp 41-86.

THERAPY

Allen W.P., and Rapp F. "Concept review of genital herpes vaccines." *Journal of Infectious Diseases* 145 (1982): 413-421.

Andrews E.B., et al. "Acyclovir in pregnancy registry: six years' experience: the acyclovir in pregnancy registry advisory committee." *Obstetrics and Gynecology* 79 (1992): 7-13.

Anonymous. "Acyclovir: a 10-year checkup." *The Helper.* American Social Health Association, Research Triangle Park, North Carolina, Fall, 1992, p. 1.

Ashley R.L., and Corey L. "effect of acyclovir treatment of primary genital herpes on the antibody response to herpes simplex virus." *Journal of Clinical Investigations* 73 (1984): 681-688.

Bernstein D.I., et al. "The effects of acyclovir on antibody response to herpes simplex virus in primary genital herpetic infections." *Journal of Infectious Diseases* 150 (1984): 7-13.

Boyd M.R., et al. "The persistent activity of BRL39123 against human herpes viruses." *Program and Abstracts of the VIIth International Congress of Virology* (August 1987).

Brown Z.A., and Watts D.H. "Antiviral therapy in pregnancy." *Clinical Obstetrics and Gynecology* 33 (1990): 276-289.

Bryson Y.J., et al. "Treatment of first episodes of genital herpes simplex virus infection with oral acyclovir: a randomized double-blind controlled trial in normal subjects." *New England Journal of Medicine* 16 (1983): 916-921.

Corey L., and Holmes K.K. "Genital herpes simplex virus infections: current concepts in diagnosis, therapy and prevention." *Annals of Internal Medicine 98* (1983): 973-983.

Douglas J.M., et al. "A double-blind study of oral acyclovir for suppression of recurrences of genital herpes simplex virus infection." *New England Journal of Medicine* 310 (1984): 1551-1556.

Elion G.B. "Mechanism of action and selectivity of acyclovir." *American Journal of Medicine* 73 (1982): 7-13.

Elion G.B., et al. "Selectivity of action of an antiherpetic agent, 9-(2-hydroxy-ethoxymethyl) guanine." *Proceedings of the National Academy of Science, USA* 74 (1977): 5716-5720.

Frenkel L.M., et al. "Pharmacokinetics of acyclovir in the term human pregnancy and neonate." *American Journal of Obstetrics and Gynecology* 164 (1991): 569-576.

Furman P.A., et al. "Metabolism of acyclovir in virus-infected and uninfected cells." *Antimicrobial Agents and Chemotherapy* 20 (1981): 518-524.

Goldberg L.H., et al. "Long-term suppression of recurrent genital herpes with acyclovir. A 5-year benchmark." *Archives of Dermatology* 129 (1993): 582-587.

Guinan M.E. "Therapy for symptomatic genital herpes simplex virus infection: a review." *Reviews of Infectious Diseases 4,* Supplement (November-December, 1982): 5819- 5828.

Kaplowitz L.G., et al. "Prolonged continuous acyclovir treatment of normal adults with frequently recurring genital herpes simplex virus infection." *Journal of the American Medical Association* 265 (1991): 747-751.

Kinghorn G.R., et al. "Acyclovir vs isoprinosine (immunovir) for suppression of recurrent genital herpes simplex infection." *Genitourinary Medicine* 68 (1992): 312-316.

Kost R.G., et al. "Recurrent acyclovir-resistant genital herpes in an immunocompetent patient." *New England Journal of Medicine* 329 (1993): 1777-1782.

Lebwohl M., et al. "Recombinant alpha-2 interferon gel treatment of recurrent herpes genitalis." *Antiviral Research* 17 (1992): 235-243.

Luby J. "Therapy in Genital Herpes." *New England Journal of Medicine,* 306 (1982): 1356-1357.

Luby J., et al. "A study of patient-initiated topical acyclovir versus placebo in the therapy of recurrent genital herpes." *Journal of Infectious Diseases* 150 (1984): 1-6.

Meier J., et al. "Immunotherapy of genital herpes with a recombinant herpes simplex virus type 2 glycoprotein D (gD2) vaccine: a placebo-controlled trial." *Clinical Research* 41 (1993): 199A.

Mertz G.J., et al. "Double-blind placebo controlled trial of oral acyclovir in first-episode genital herpes simplex virus infection." *Journal of the American Medical Association* 252 (1984): 1147-1151.

Mindel A., et al. "Prophylactic oral acyclovir in recurrent genital herpes." *The Lancet II* (1984): 57-59.

Reichman R.C., et al. "Treatment of recurrent genital herpes simplex infections with oral acyclovir. a controlled trial." *Journal of the American Medical Association* 251 (1984): 2103-2117.

Sacks S.L. "The role of oral acyclovir in the management of genital herpes simplex." *Canadian Medical Association Journal* 136 (1987): 701-707.

Sacks S.L., et al. "Randomized, double-blind, placebo-controlled, clinic-initiated, Canadian, multicenter study of topical 3% edoxudine cream in the treatment of recurrent genital herpes." *Journal of Infectious Diseases* 164 (1991): 665-672.

Sacks S.L., et al. "Randomized, double-blind, placebo-controlled, patient-initiated study of topical high- and low-dose alpha interferon with nonoxynol-9 in the treatment of recurrent genital herpes." *Journal of Infectious Diseases* 161 (1990): 692-698.

Sacks S.L., et al. "Chronic suppression for six months compared with intermittent lesional therapy of frequently recurring genital herpes using oral acyclovir: effects on lesions and nonlesional prodromes." *Sexually Transmitted Diseases* 15(1988): 58-62.

Safrin S., et al. "A controlled trial comparing foscarnet with vidarabine for acyclovir-resistant mucocutaneous herpes simplex in the acquired immunodeficiency syndrome." *New England Journal of Medicine* 325 (1991): 551-555.

Shupack J., et al. "Topical alpha-interferon ointment with dimethyl sulfoxide in the treatment of recurrent genital herpes simplex." *Dermatology* 184 (1992): 40-44.

Skinner G.R., et al. "Report of twelve years experience in open study of Skinner herpes simplex vaccine towards prevention of herpes genitalis." *Medical Microbiology and Immunology* (Berlin) 180 (1992): 305-320.

Straus E.E., et al. "Suppression of frequently recurring genital herpes: a placebo-controlled double-blind trial of oral acyclovir." *New England Journal of Medicine* 310 (1984): 1545-1550.

Whitley R.J., and Gnann, J.W. Jr. "Acyclovir: a decade later." *New England Journal of Medicine* 327 (1992): 782-789.

Wise T.G., et al. "Herpes simplex vaccines." *Journal of Infectious Diseases* 136 (1977): 706-710.

Viridae Herpes Clinic History Form

This is a medical history form similar to the one we give to patients at the Viridae Clinical Sciences Herpes Clinic. You may find it useful to read this to see what types of information you may want to think about when going to your health care provider. The latter sections contain questions for pregnant and non-pregnant women. Feel free to photocopy and fill out this form before you go to your health care provider. This would be one way to provide the most important information about your herpes and about your medical and sexual history.

The following history form is designed for you to fill out either in the clinic or before your visit. Please spend the time to carefully answer the questions. The purpose of the form is to give your physician your full history so that nothing important is missed, while also recognizing that much of what you are here for may be counseling and discussion. The nurse and physician will go over this form with you. Please bring it with you. If you are uncomfortable answering some of the questions, please refuse to answer those specific questions and fill in the rest.

Within the law, all information concerning any part of your medical care will be held in the strictest confidence, unless you specifically consent or ask us, in writing, to release specific information (e.g., if you move and want your new physician to have a record from us). Because of what we do here, we are, of course, especially concerned about personal privacy matters. Nevertheless, it is our legal and medical responsibility to keep a record of your visit here. Our clinic charts are not part of the regular hospital medical record system, although any specimens obtained from you as part of your examination may be sent to a licensed medical laboratory for a test. Your physician or nurse will be happy to explain to you any aspects of this form or the clinic process which you do not understand. As a normal part of the assessment here, you should expect that the physician will want to talk with you fully about your concerns. Please feel free to bring someone with you into the interview if you wish. If you want your partner with you, please let us know this before your interview.

Expect your physician, as a part of the normal process, to perform a full physical examination. If you prefer a female attendant (chaperone) present during your examination, one will be provided. If you do not wish to be examined at all, however, bring this fact immediately to the attention of someone from the clinic so that alternate arrangements can be made. Thank you.

Name

_____

Date of birth

_____
(day/month/year)

What is the date you are filling out this form?

_____
(day/month/year)

During the physical examination—
is an attendant requested?

_____ Yes   _____ No

Signed

_____

Current Marital Status

_____ Never married   _____ Divorced   _____ Widowed

_____ Married   _____ Separated   _____ Common-law

Have you been married more than one time?

_____ Yes   _____ No

If so how many times have you been married?

   1   2   3   4   5

How would you describe your racial background?

_____ Caucasian   _____ Other Asian

_____ Chinese   _____ Black   _____ Other

What is your occupation?

_____

_____

Substance History

Have you ever smoked regularly?

_____ Yes   _____ No

Do you currently smoke regularly?

_____ Yes   _____ No

How many cigarettes do you/did you smoke daily?

_____

For a total of how many years have you/did you smoke?

_____

Approximately how much per week do you consume of the following?

Liquor (no. of mixed or straight drinks)   _____ Drinks per week

Wine (glasses of wine)   _____ Glasses per week

Beer (bottles of beer)   _____ Bottles per week

Have you ever used drugs by injection with a needle?

_____ Yes   _____ No

If yes, last date used

_____
(day/month/year)

Do you currently use drugs by injection with a needle?

_____ Yes   _____ No

Other than alcohol and cigarettes, list other drugs you may have used for
recreational purposes:

_____

295

If listed, last date used

_____
(day/month/year)

Past Medical History

Have you had any serious past medical illness not yet described?
Please describe:

_____

Have you had any minor or major surgery not yet described?
Please describe:

_____

Current medical history (not necessarily related to herpes)

Have you been suffering from any of the following problems lately?
(please indicate with a check mark (√) in the appropriate space.)

_____ Unexplained weight changes
_____ Waking up during the night
_____ Poor appetite
_____ Waking up earlier than you should
_____ Fevers
_____ Difficulty falling to sleep
_____ Frequent sweats at night which wet the sheets
_____ A feeling the world would be better off without you
_____ Chills
_____ Swallowed food sticking in the throat or chest
_____ Cough productive of sputum from the chest
_____ Heartburn
_____ Cough with blood
_____ Nausea or vomiting
_____ Noises when you breathe (wheeze)
_____ Hemorrhoids
_____ Lump in your breast(s)
_____ Pain in your abdomen
_____ Chest pain
_____ Swelling of your ankles
_____ Unexplained bruising or bleeding
_____ Diarrhea or constipation
_____ Tired more often than you should be
_____ Fatigued by activities you shouldn't be

_____ Much hotter or colder than others with you

_____ General loss of energy

_____ Uncontrollable bouts of hunger or thirst

_____ So drained that you cannot move

_____ Visual difficulty not corrected by glasses

_____ Problems with your ability to concentrate

_____ Frequent headaches

_____ Problems making decisions

_____ Persistent difficulty with hearing

_____ A feeling of pain or tenderness in the muscles

_____ Changes in your voice

_____ Sleep disturbance

_____ Problems with your teeth or gums

_____ A sense of worthlessness

_____ Irregular beating of your heart (palpitations)

_____ A sense of guilt

_____ Blood clots (phlebitis)

_____ Swollen glands or nodes in the neck

_____ Fainting or blacking out

_____ Tender glands or nodes in the neck

_____ Getting up at night to urinate more than once

_____ A feeling of weakness in the muscles

_____ Loss of pleasure in things

_____ Excessive moodiness or black moods

_____ Loss of interest in things

_____ A feeling of being depressed

_____ Thinking a lot about death

_____ Thoughts about suicide

_____ A feeling of pain or tenderness in the joints (knees, ankles, wrists, etc.)

(Please indicate with a check mark (√) in the appropriate space.)

Have you ever?   If yes, approximate date

_____ Had an ulcer   _____

_____ Vomited blood   _____

_____ Had a transfusion of blood   _____
       or any blood products

_____ Had yellow skin (jaundice)   _____

_____ Had hepatitis   _____

Have you ever?   If yes, approximate date

_____ Had blood in your bowel movements   _____

_____ Had blood in your urine   _____

_____ Had urine brown like the
         color of Coca Cola®   _____

_____ Had kidney stones   _____

_____ Had a urinary tract infection
         (bladder or kidney)   _____

_____ Had problems with your joints   _____

_____ Had a skin condition   _____

_____ Had eczema   _____

_____ Had a tremor
         (uncontrollable shaking of your hands) _____

_____ Had gonorrhea   _____

_____ Had genital warts   _____

_____ Had pelvic inflamitory disease (PID)   _____

_____ Had trichomonas infection   _____

_____ Had chlamydia infection   _____

_____ Had syphllis   _____

Family History

Father: _____ Alive   _____ His current age

                     _____ Deceased   _____ His age at the
                                                   time of death

Diseases he has (or had during his life)

_____

_____

Appendix 3: Viridae Herpes Clinic History Form

Mother: _____ Alive   _____ Her current age

                         _____ Deceased   _____ Her age at the time of death

Diseases she has (or had during her life)

_____

_____

Siblings

    List ages of all of your living brothers

_____

    List ages of all of your living sisters

_____

    List ages at death of deceased brothers

_____

    List ages at death of deceased sisters

_____

    List significant diseases in your sisters or brothers

_____

_____

    List significant diseases running in your family

_____

_____

Sexual History

At what age did you first have intimate sexual contact?
(e.g. vaginal or anal intercourse, or oral/genital contact etc.)

_____ Years old

Approximately how many different sexual partners have you had
in the past 2 weeks?

0   1   2   3   4   6   7   8   9   10

Approximately how many different sexual partners have you had
in the past 6 months?

0   1   2   3   4   6   7   8   9   10 or more

Approximately how many different sexual partners have you had
in the past 2 years?

0   1   2   3   4   6   7   8   9   10   11   12   13   14   15   16   17   18   19   20 or more

Approximately how many different sexual partners have
you had in your entire lifetime?

0   1   2   3   4   6   7   8   9   10   11   12   13   14   15   16   17   18   19   20

21   22   23   24   25   26   27   28   29   30   31   32   33   34   35   36   37   38   39   40

41   42   43   44   45   46   47   48   49   50   51   52   53   54   55   56   57   58   59   60

If more, how many? _____

Have you had sex with another member of the same sex?

_____ Frequently   _____ Occasionally   _____ Never

How would you describe your sexual preference?

_____ Heterosexual   _____ Homosexual   _____ Bisexual

Do you practice safer sex currently?

_____ Always   _____ Occasionally   _____ Never

Remember that you are not compelled to answer any question on this form.
Refusing to answer will not prejudice your care in any way.

300

Have you ever been tested for HIV (AIDS)?

_____ Yes   _____ No

If yes, when was the most recent test?

_____
(day/month/year)

If yes, what was the most recent test result?

_____ Positive   _____ Negative

Herpes History

Do you think that you have ever had genital herpes?

_____ Yes   _____ No   _____ Maybe

Do you think that you have ever had anal herpes?

_____ Yes   _____ No   _____ Maybe

Do you think that you have ever had lip herpes (cold sores)?

_____ Yes   _____ No   _____ Maybe

If applicable to you:
When did you first get symptoms of genital or anal herpes?

_____
(day/month/year)

How long did your first outbreak of genital herpes take to heal completely?

_____ Days

Was your first outbreak of genital herpes much different from subsequent ones?

_____ Much worse   _____ Much less severe

_____ Slightly worse   _____ Slightly less severe

_____ Same

THE TRUTH ABOUT HERPES

The average number of separate herpes recurrences you experience during an average month is:

0   1/2   1   2   3   4   6   7   8   9

The approximate number of separate herpes recurrences you experienced during the last 6 months was:

0   1   2   3   4   6   7   8   9   10 or more

The approximate number of separate herpes recurrences you experienced during the last 12 months was:

0   1   2   3   4   6   7   8   9   10   11   12   13   14   15   16 or more

_____ If more than 16, how many?

Approximately how many separate outbreaks of genital herpes have you ever had?

_____ outbreaks

Since your first experience with herpes, do you feel the frequency of outbreaks has:

_____ Increased   _____ Decreased   _____ Stayed the same

From start of warning to total healing, how long does each recurrence usually last in days?

0   1   2   3   4   6   7   8   9

If more than 9, how many days? _____

What was the date of your last herpes outbreak?

_____
(day/month/year)

Are you having an outbreak or warning today?

_____ Yes   _____ No

Appendix 3: Viridae Herpes Clinic History Form

Please indicate with a check mark (√) in the appropriate space.

How was your herpes diagnosed?

_____ Viral culture. if yes, date obtained:

_____

(day/month/year)

Lab name _____

_____ Physician opinion (no test)

_____ Blood test; Explain:_____

_____

_____ My opinion (no test)

_____ Other

Which of the following trigger your herpes outbreaks?

_____ Menses   _____ Emotional stress

_____ Sexual contact _____ Medicine

_____ Weather   _____ Sunlight

_____ Fever   _____ Other

Have you discussed your herpes with a sexual partner?

_____ Every time before beginning a new sexual intimacy

_____ Every time after beginning a new sexual intimacy

_____ Yes, with some partners, but not all

_____ Never

_____ Not applicable

What are your greatest concerns about having herpes?

_____

_____

_____

_____

Have you ever transmitted herpes to a sexual partner that you know of?

_____ Yes   _____ No   _____ Not Applicable
(no new sexual partner
since getting herpes)

What are the usual characteristics of a herpes recurrence for you?

_____ Warning first
_____ Sores hurt
_____ Sores itch
_____ Sores tingle
_____ Sores burn
_____ Sores are tender to touch
_____ Urination hurts
_____ Vaginal discharge
_____ Lymph nodes in the groin enlarge and hurt
_____ Fever
_____ Headache
_____ Stiff neck
_____ Rectal pain
_____ Rectal itch
_____ Sore throat
_____ Muscle aches
_____ Leg pain
_____ Buttock pain
_____ Constipation
_____ Altered mood or emotions

Medication History

Have you ever taken an oral antiviral drug (acyclovir [Zovirax®], famciclovir [Famvir®], valacyclovir [Valtrex®]) to suppress outbreaks?

_____ Yes   _____ No   Drug used

_____

Appendix 3: Viridae Herpes Clinic History Form

Has suppression with oral antiviral drugs been effective?

_____ Yes _____ No

Have you taken an oral antiviral drug to suppress outbreaks in the past year?

_____ Yes _____ No

If yes, how many outbreaks did you have in the 6 months just before starting?

_____

If yes, how many outbreaks did you have in the 12 months just before starting?

_____

If yes, when did you last take a daily oral antiviral drug for suppression?

Start date	Stop date	Drug used
_____	_____	_____
(day/month/year)	(day/month/year)	

Have you stopped taking an oral antiviral drug to suppress outbreaks?

_____ Yes _____ No

If yes, how many outbreaks have you had since stopping an oral antiviral drug?

_____

If no (i.e., you are still taking it), how many outbreaks have you had in the past 6 months?

_____

Have you ever taken an oral antiviral drug to treat an individual outbreak?

_____ Yes _____ No

Has treatment of individual outbreaks with an oral antiviral drug been effective?

_____ Yes _____ No

Last dates of intermittent oral antiviral drug use to treat individual episodes (starting from most recent).

Start date   Stop date   Drug used

_____   _____   _____
(day/month/year)   (day/month/year)

Start date   Stop date   Drug used

_____   _____   _____
(day/month/year)   (day/month/year)

Start date   Stop date   Drug used

_____   _____   _____
(day/month/year)   (day/month/year)

Start date   Stop date   Drug used

_____   _____   _____
(day/month/year)   (day/month/year)

Have you ever used topical acyclovir (Zovirax®) ointment?

_____ Yes   _____ No

Are you currently using topical acyclovir (Zovirax®) ointment?

_____ Yes   _____ No

Has topical acyclovir (Zovirax®) been effective?

_____ Yes   _____ No

Have you ever used topical edoxudine (Virostat®) ointment?

_____ Yes   _____ No

Are you currently using topical edoxudine (Virostat®) ointment?

_____ Yes   _____ No

Has topical edoxudine (Virostat®) been effective?

_____ Yes   _____ No

Are you presently taking medication prescribed by a physician or purchased "over the counter" for any medical problem, herpes or otherwise, including aspirin, vitamins, lysine, antacids, etc? If yes, please state name and dosage. Please bring medication with you.

_____

Have you ever been allergic to any medication (e.g., penicillin) or other specific item?

_____ Yes   _____ No

If yes, describe:

_____

_____

(List all allergies if applicable: including food, dust, pollens, etc.)

Menstrual/Obstetric History

What was the date of your last normal menstrual period?

_____
(day/month/year)

What was the date of your last PAP test?

_____
(day/month/year)

Do you have a history of abnormal PAP tests?

_____ Yes   _____ No   _____ Unknown

Do you have bothersome vaginal discharge?

_____ Yes   _____ No

How old were you when you had your first menstrual period?

_____ years old

Have you ever been pregnant?

_____ Yes   _____ No

How many times have you been pregnant in your lifetime?

0   1   2   3   4   6   7   8   9   10 or more

If so, how old were you when you *first* became pregnant?

_____ years old

How many children have you had?

    0 1 2 3 4 6 7 8 9 10 or more

How many children with health problems have you had?

    0 1 2 3 4 6 7 8 9 10 or more

How many children born prematurely have you had?

    0 1 2 3 4 6 7 8 9 10 or more

How many cesarean sections have you had in your lifetime?

    0 1 2 3 4 6 7 8 9 10 or more

How many therapeutic abortions have you had in your lifetime?

    0 1 2 3 4 6 7 8 9 10 or more

Pregnancy History

Have you had a test for German measles (rubella)?

_____ Yes   _____ No

Have you had a vaccination for rubella?

_____ Yes   _____ No

What is your current week of pregnancy (gestation)?

_____ Weeks

What is your expected date of confinement (delivery)?

_____
(day/month/year)

Have you had an ultrasound?

_____ Yes   _____ No

Have you had any bleeding or spotting from the vagina during this pregnancy?

_____ Yes   _____ No

Thank you for taking the time to fill out this questionnaire.

Index

Order Form

If you cannot obtain a copy of this book from a bookstore or health clinic, you may order a copy from the publisher by using this order form or calling (604) 922-6588.

We also supply multiple copies of this book to bookstores and health clinics world wide; please contact us for information on discounts.

Name _____

Address _____

_____

Country _____ Postal code _____

Please send me _____ copies of *The Truth About Herpes* by Stephen L. Sacks, M.D.

Total amount enclosed _____

☐ Cheque/money order enclosed, payable to

Gordon Soules Book Publishers Ltd.

☐ Visa ☐ MasterCard ☐ American Express

Card no. _____ Expiry date _____

In the United States and other countries outside Canada, return this form to:

Gordon Soules Book Publishers Ltd.
620—1916 Pike Place
Seattle, WA 98101, USA
Fax: (604) 688-5442   E-mail: books@gordonsoules.com
Web site: http://www.gordonsoules.com

Price per copy: $24.95 (U.S. funds)
Add postage and handling:
United States: $5.00 first book, $1.00 each additional book (surface mail)
Outside the United States and Canada: $14.00 first book,
$8.00 each additional book (air mail)

In Canada, return this form to:

Gordon Soules Book Publishers Ltd.
1354-B Marine Drive
West Vancouver, BC V7T 1B5
Fax: (604) 688-5442   E-mail: books@gordonsoules.com
Web site: http://www.gordonsoules.com

Price per copy: $26.70 ($24.95 plus $1.75 GST)
Add postage and handling: $5.35 ($5.00 plus 35¢ GST) first book,
$1.07 ($1.00 plus 7¢ GST) each additional book (surface mail)

CUT HERE

Order Form

If you cannot obtain a copy of this book from a bookstore or health clinic, you may order a copy from the publisher by using this order form or calling (604) 922-6588.

We also supply multiple copies of this book to bookstores and health clinics world wide; please contact us for information on discounts.

Name _____

Address _____

_____

Country _____ Postal code _____

Please send me _____ copies of *The Truth About Herpes* by Stephen L. Sacks, M.D.

Total amount enclosed _____

☐ Cheque/money order enclosed, payable to

Gordon Soules Book Publishers Ltd.

☐ Visa ☐ MasterCard ☐ American Express

Card no. _____ Expiry date _____

In the United States and other countries outside Canada, return this form to:

Gordon Soules Book Publishers Ltd.
620—1916 Pike Place
Seattle, WA 98101, USA
Fax: (604) 688-5442 E-mail: books@gordonsoules.com
Web site: http://www.gordonsoules.com

Price per copy: $24.95 (U.S. funds)
Add postage and handling:
United States: $5.00 first book, $1.00 each additional book (surface mail)
Outside the United States and Canada: $14.00 first book,
$8.00 each additional book (air mail)

In Canada, return this form to:

Gordon Soules Book Publishers Ltd.
1354-B Marine Drive
West Vancouver, BC V7T 1B5
Fax: (604) 688-5442 E-mail: books@gordonsoules.com
Web site: http://www.gordonsoules.com

Price per copy: $26.70 ($24.95 plus $1.75 GST)
Add postage and handling: $5.35 ($5.00 plus 35¢ GST) first book,
$1.07 ($1.00 plus 7¢ GST) each additional book (surface mail)

Order Form

If you cannot obtain a copy of this book from a bookstore or health clinic, you may order a copy from the publisher by using this order form or calling (604) 922-6588.

We also supply multiple copies of this book to bookstores and health clinics world wide; please contact us for information on discounts.

Name _____

Address _____

_____

Country _____ Postal code _____

Please send me _____ copies of *The Truth About Herpes* by Stephen L. Sacks, M.D.

Total amount enclosed _____

☐ Cheque/money order enclosed, payable to

Gordon Soules Book Publishers Ltd.

☐ Visa   ☐ MasterCard   ☐ American Express

Card no. _____ Expiry date _____

In the United States and other countries outside Canada, return this form to:

Gordon Soules Book Publishers Ltd.
620—1916 Pike Place
Seattle, WA 98101, USA
Fax: (604) 688-5442   E-mail: books@gordonsoules.com
Web site: http://www.gordonsoules.com

Price per copy: $24.95 (U.S. funds)
Add postage and handling:
United States: $5.00 first book, $1.00 each additional book (surface mail)
Outside the United States and Canada: $14.00 first book,
$8.00 each additional book (air mail)

In Canada, return this form to:

Gordon Soules Book Publishers Ltd.
1354-B Marine Drive
West Vancouver, BC V7T 1B5
Fax: (604) 688-5442   E-mail: books@gordonsoules.com
Web site: http://www.gordonsoules.com

Price per copy: $26.70 ($24.95 plus $1.75 GST)
Add postage and handling: $5.35 ($5.00 plus 35¢ GST) first book,
$1.07 ($1.00 plus 7¢ GST) each additional book (surface mail)

CUT HERE

Order Form

If you cannot obtain a copy of this book from a bookstore or health clinic, you may order a copy from the publisher by using this order form or calling (604) 922-6588.

We also supply multiple copies of this book to bookstores and health clinics world wide; please contact us for information on discounts.

Name _____

Address _____

_____

Country _____ Postal code _____

Please send me _____ copies of *The Truth About Herpes* by Stephen L. Sacks, M.D.

Total amount enclosed _____

☐ Cheque/money order enclosed, payable to

Gordon Soules Book Publishers Ltd.

☐ Visa ☐ MasterCard ☐ American Express

Card no. _____ Expiry date _____

In the United States and other countries outside Canada, return this form to:

Gordon Soules Book Publishers Ltd.
620—1916 Pike Place
Seattle, WA 98101, USA
Fax: (604) 688-5442   E-mail: books@gordonsoules.com
Web site: http://www.gordonsoules.com

Price per copy: $24.95 (U.S. funds)
Add postage and handling:
United States: $5.00 first book, $1.00 each additional book (surface mail)
Outside the United States and Canada: $14.00 first book,
$8.00 each additional book (air mail)

In Canada, return this form to:

Gordon Soules Book Publishers Ltd.
1354-B Marine Drive
West Vancouver, BC V7T 1B5
Fax: (604) 688-5442   E-mail: books@gordonsoules.com
Web site: http://www.gordonsoules.com

Price per copy: $26.70 ($24.95 plus $1.75 GST)
Add postage and handling: $5.35 ($5.00 plus 35¢ GST) first book,
$1.07 ($1.00 plus 7¢ GST) each additional book (surface mail)

CUT HERE

Order Form

If you cannot obtain a copy of this book from a bookstore or health clinic, you may order a copy from the publisher by using this order form or calling (604) 922-6588.

We also supply multiple copies of this book to bookstores and health clinics world wide; please contact us for information on discounts.

Name _____

Address _____

_____

Country _____ Postal code _____

Please send me _____ copies of *The Truth About Herpes* by Stephen L. Sacks, M.D.

Total amount enclosed _____

☐ Cheque/money order enclosed, payable to

Gordon Soules Book Publishers Ltd.

☐ Visa   ☐ MasterCard   ☐ American Express

Card no. _____ Expiry date _____

In the United States and other countries outside Canada, return this form to:

Gordon Soules Book Publishers Ltd.
620—1916 Pike Place
Seattle, WA 98101, USA
Fax: (604) 688-5442   E-mail: books@gordonsoules.com
Web site: http://www.gordonsoules.com

Price per copy: $24.95 (U.S. funds)
Add postage and handling:
United States: $5.00 first book, $1.00 each additional book (surface mail)
Outside the United States and Canada: $14.00 first book,
$8.00 each additional book (air mail)

In Canada, return this form to:

Gordon Soules Book Publishers Ltd.
1354-B Marine Drive
West Vancouver, BC V7T 1B5
Fax: (604) 688-5442   E-mail: books@gordonsoules.com
Web site: http://www.gordonsoules.com

Price per copy: $26.70 ($24.95 plus $1.75 GST)
Add postage and handling: $5.35 ($5.00 plus 35¢ GST) first book,
$1.07 ($1.00 plus 7¢ GST) each additional book (surface mail)